SPE

The Marv

"*The Marvelous Transformation* is an engaging testament to the power of taking responsibility for your own well-being. Pain is unavoidable, but suffering is a choice. With unflinching honesty, Emily Filmore instructs and inspires by her own courageous example, showing readers how to transcend the pain and frustration of living with a chronic illness to live a life of joy, purpose, and deep personal satisfaction. I highly recommend this compassionate guide to anyone suffering from an autoimmune disease who is interested in dramatically increasing their quality of life."

Terry Wahls, MD
CLINICAL PROFESSOR OF INTERNAL MEDICINE, UNIVERSITY OF IOWA
Author of The Wahls Protocol: A Radical New Way to Treat All Chronic Autoimmune Conditions Using Paleo Principles

"*The Marvelous Transformation* is an honest, intimate, and entertaining read based on personal experience with autoimmunity. Emily engages her readers by incorporating activities throughout the book while guiding them through their exploration into a complex illness process that does not have to be a negative experience. Whether you are a patient, caregiver, healthcare professional, or interested in learning more about living with autoimmunity, you will find great knowledge, an array of resources, and helpful tips that you will want to share with your family and friends to help them better understand autoimmunity.

Jerry Williams
BOARD PRESIDENT · *Myositis Support and Understanding Association*

"A must-read for autoimmune patients. A delightful book that empowers you and those who love you to make the best out of a difficult relationship with autoimmune disease. This book will help you find your healthfulness."

Patricia Barber
ASSISTANT DIRECTOR AND PATIENT EDUCATOR
American Autoimmune Related Diseases Association

"Emily Filmore writes about her struggle with autoimmune disease with honesty and compassion. She offers tips on how to thrive while living with physical limitations that come straight from her own experience. If you or someone you love suffers from an autoimmune disease, Emily's words will help you feel less alone in what often feels like a lonely grind."

Aisha Sultan
NATIONALLY SYNDICATED, AWARD-WINNING COLUMNIST
Home and Family Editor for the St. Louis Post-Dispatch

"In the US alone, it is estimated that one in five or 20 percent of people suffer from autoimmune diseases. Emily Filmore lovingly and openly shares her journey—one of learning, spirituality, strength, love, and compassion. This book is bound to help others by inspiring them, and their family members, to know they too can handle anything that life might throw at them."

Karin Volo
Best-selling author of Engage! *and the* Bringing Joy *series*

THE
Marvelous Transformation

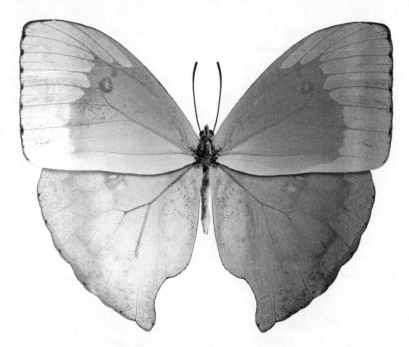

THE
Marvelous
Transformation

Living Well with Autoimmune Disease

EMILY A. FILMORE

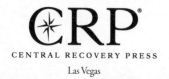

CENTRAL RECOVERY PRESS

Las Vegas

Central Recovery Press (CRP) is committed to publishing exceptional materials addressing addiction treatment, recovery, and behavioral healthcare topics, including original and quality books, audio/visual communications, and web-based new media. Through a diverse selection of titles, we seek to contribute a broad range of unique resources for professionals, recovering individuals and their families, and the general public.

For more information, visit www.centralrecoverypress.com.

Publisher: Central Recovery Press
           3321 N. Buffalo Drive
           Las Vegas, NV 89129

20 19 18 17 16 15   1 2 3 4 5

ISBN: 978-1-937612-87-0 (paper)
      978-1-937612-88-7 (e-book)

Photo of Emily A. Filmore by David Soto, Jr.

Publisher's Note: This book contains general information about autoimmune disease and related chronic illnesses. The information is not medical advice, and should not be treated as such. Central Recovery Press makes no representations or warranties in relation to the information in this book. If you have any specific questions about any medical matter discussed in this book, you should consult your doctor or other professional healthcare provider. This book is not an alternative to medical advice from your doctor or other professional healthcare provider.

Our books represent the experiences and opinions of their authors only. Every effort has been made to ensure that events, institutions, and statistics presented in our books as facts are accurate and up-to-date. To protect their privacy, the names of some of the people, places, and institutions in this book may have been changed.

Cover and interior design by Marisa Jackson

Scott, our love is infinite;
I am grateful for each day with you.
Sage and Rickey, you give me laughter,
joy, and a desire to keep fighting.

Table of Contents

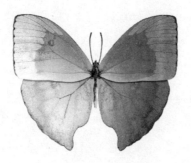

FOREWORD

You are about to read one of the most inspiring, practical, and helpful books you could ever hope to lay your hands on. It is a book about an autoimmune disease, yet it is not about a specific illness so much as it is about a specific kind of healthfulness.

Emily's story is a striking and encouraging example of how anyone can be mentally, emotionally, and spiritually healthy, even as they are physically unhealthy. This is a powerful kind of healthfulness that can even minimize the effects of physical disease. That is, it can be the greatest healing device, the greatest medicine, of all.

Yes, we've heard this before, but here is a living, breathing example of it that makes real all that we've been told about the power of the mind and spirit. These pages demonstrate the strength of the human spirit in the face of enormous challenges, the capacity of humor to transform difficult circumstances, and the immense resource that a partnership with the soul can provide to the body and the mind in the most testing situations.

You'll find plenty of smiles and a few out-loud laughs here, along with a list of remarkably useful tools and strategies for dealing with a health condition that receives little attention by the national fundraising community, but which profoundly affects the day-to-day lives of millions of people.

My life has been deeply enriched by knowing Emily personally. She stands as a continual inspiration to me, and I am grateful to her for sharing her experience in such a personal way. It has given me strength as I meet the tests and trials of my own life. I know her story can affect you in the same way. On behalf of all of us, *thank you,* Emily Filmore, for your transformative transparency. We are blessed in you.

Neale Donald Walsch
New York Times *best-selling author*
of Conversations with God

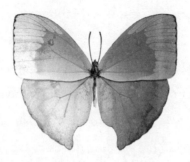

ACKNOWLEDGMENTS

To Neale Donald Walsch: This book would not exist were it not for you, your mentoring, and your encouragement. Your work inspires me and our friendship warms my heart.

To Scott: Your dedication to this project has been inexhaustible. Thank you for reading the manuscript countless times, for allowing me to wake you in the middle of the night to rework a passage, and for always being you, my perfect companion.

To Rickey and Sage: The light and humor in our home is evident in the pages of this book. Thank you for your patience in dealing with a lack of groceries, a messy house, and my long hours of introspection.

To Mary and Dave Meehan, Tom and Marti Boling, and Jane Filmore: Your belief in me is unmatched. Your parental love and support gave me the courage to share this story.

To Drew, Laura, Lucas, Wendee, Grandma, Yvonne, Jaime, Amy C., Jon, Katie, Amy B., Laurie—all of my family members and friends: You have cheered me on, listened to me cry, helped me laugh, dissected details, read drafts, and always had my back. My life is made better by you, as is this book.

To Jaye Schnell, Bob Hansen, Wayne Zade, and Carl Helfrich: You, my most treasured teachers, helped shape who I am today. Each of you in your own ways have instilled in me a love of learning, the ability and desire to help people, the enjoyment of writing, and the skill of expressing myself more efficiently. I hope you find your hearts and souls reflected within these pages.

To Jami Lynn Sands: Your invaluable advice and expertise will help ensure my message goes far.

To Bill Gladstone: Thank you for finding the right publisher at the right time to get this work out into the world. I am forever grateful for your efforts.

To Central Recovery Press—the entire editing, design, and marketing team, and especially my editor, Eliza Tutellier: Thank you for believing in my story, and in my vision of hope and transformation. Your guidance has been invaluable.

And lastly, to Autoimmunity: Thank you for your gifts. I may not have chosen you, but I believe you and I are making the best of a difficult relationship.

You Can Heal Your Disease and It Can Heal You

"The concept 'you create your own reality' is the single most dangerous idea in spirituality today."

The speaker was Neale Donald Walsch, the *New York Times* best-selling author on spirituality. I was sitting in Neale's family room for a three-day brainstorming and writing session when he asked me how I was doing. Not in the passing sense as you might ask a friend on the street, but "How are you *doing?*" with emphasis on the "doing."

I had been working for him for nearly three years, so he knew I had an autoimmune disease. He also knew I had almost missed this trip to his house due to multiple back-to-back infections.

As I launched into how I was *doing,* he stopped me and asked me to start from the beginning. He asked me to tell him how I became sick, what my exact diagnosis was, and what "they" were doing to help me. He wanted to hear the whole story.

An autoimmune disease can be loosely described as any one of numerous types of hypersensitivity or inappropriate immune responses the body has to substances normally present in the body itself. It is, in brief, an attack *by* the body *on* the body and is not fun.

Over eighty illnesses are caused by autoimmunity, and if you have any one of them (a significant portion of the population does), you know it. You certainly know you are miserable a lot of the time, even if you don't know to call it an autoimmune disease.

When I was done telling Neale about all of this, he said, "Wow, you could write a book about that, and it would probably help a lot of people."

It had never occurred to me that my disease could be of help to someone else. What I do know is that I would have given my eye teeth for a book on what I've been going through these past decades . . . something that would have told me what was going on, why it was happening, and how I should deal with it—even how I could celebrate it. Because now, after many years of struggle and suffering, I do experience my autoimmune disease as a springboard to personal happiness.

Yes, I said it: *happiness.*

Not Making Light of Disease

Diseases caused by autoimmunity are often chronic and can be debilitating and sometimes even life-threatening, so I don't mean to make light of them. Nevertheless, they don't have to rob us of the good and the wonderful, the joyful, and the meaningful aspects of life—quite the opposite, in fact. They can be the very impetus that throws open the door to such experiences.

I assume you were drawn to this book because you are dealing with some form of an autoimmune disease, either personally or as someone who loves and supports a person with such an illness. If so, and if you've been searching for this kind of book—one with the insight and support only a person who is walking the same path could offer—I am so glad you have arrived here.

Some parts of my story may seem depressing. I include those parts not to scare you but to show you that someone has been there before you. The severity of symptoms differs for every patient, and there are many who struggle with more than what I am experiencing. Undoubtedly, you will recognize part of your own story within my descriptions and realize that you're neither alone nor crazy. My aim is to uplift you, to provide you with relief, and to show you that you do not have to allow the disease to rule your life.

Finding Divinity

I use the words "divinity" and "God" interchangeably, and I want to clarify what I mean. I don't adhere to any particular spiritual belief or practice but have created my own eclectic set of ideas about life and the soul's place in the universe based on readings in various philosophies, including new age spirituality, Buddhism,

Hinduism, and ancient Indian spirituality. I believe each of our souls is a spark of love—an equal, creative member of the collective intelligence that comprises the universe—and that we are each an indivisible part of what some people call God.

When I discuss "finding divinity," I am referring to a transcendent moment of pure peace, love, joy, and perfection: the chance to feel oneness with God, the universe, and all of humanity. It is in these profound moments of bliss, despite my physical limitations, that I encounter true happiness and experience the magic of living well. No matter your own spiritual or religious belief, I trust you will substitute a word or phrase of your liking whenever I say "divinity"; it might be "happiness," "peace," "love," "clarity," "forgiveness," "grace," "growth," "truth," "source," or "God." What matters is that you find that life-affirming feeling of peace within your own experience and understanding.

Your Experience Can Be Healed

Let's now look at this experience you are having and explore ways to heal it—not necessarily the disease itself, but the difficulties you may be having related to it.

I'm inviting you on a journey of introspection, self-discovery, awakening, and growth. By sharing my own experiences, I hope to provide you with a mirror for your own. As I wrote about my life, I laughed and experienced moments of exhilaration but also moments of excruciating, if cathartic, emotional pain. Those moments, sobbing and rocking on the floor, furthered my own transformation, a process that is ongoing. In sharing my story I further healed myself. And this is the lesson I hope to pass on to you.

Each chapter focuses on a particular aspect of living with an autoimmune disease. As each chapter begins, I invite you to "Take Stock of Where You Are Now" through questions, prompts, and suggestions for you to write about in a journal. At the end of each chapter, I provide you with additional and complementary questions, prompts, and suggestions to help you "Create Your Own Marvelous Transformation." These journaling prompts challenge you to realize where you are right now; to process what you have read; to think deeply about how it applies to your life; and to positively transform your own thoughts, beliefs, and feelings about your health.

In addition to the story of my own experiences and the journaling prompts, I include three sections in each chapter that are carefully designed to help you get the most out of the book. They are "The Wonderful Pieces of Divinity I Have Found," "Creative Tips for Empowering Yourself," and "Caregiver Tips." "The Wonderful Pieces of Divinity I Have Found" are the quick little tidbits you can refer to that encapsulate the glimpses of the divine I've been given; they are my recipe of coping skills with which to find happiness in the face of my disease. "Creative Tips for Empowering Yourself" include exercises designed to lead you to your own sense of well-being. "Caregiver Tips" are ideas for significant others of autoimmunity patients that I believe will make life easier for both of you.

Armed with the knowledge presented in this book, I invite you to write the story of your own *Marvelous Transformation*. Let this book guide you as you embrace your feelings, allowing yourself to look closely at the realities of living with a chronic disease. Let it help you realize and choose what kind of life you want to lead, in spite of your health.

I don't live every day in utter bliss. I do get mad, sad, and lose hope just like everyone else. However, those moments are fleeting because a long time ago I chose—and I continue to choose—to live, love, and laugh my way through this illness. By remembering, reliving, and sharing these crucial moments of my life, I hope to inspire you and to help you find your own peace and happiness.

Create Your Own Marvelous Transformation

1. Grab a notebook, a journal, or any old pen and paper. At the top of the page, write a heading with the date and your name with the words "Marvelous Transformation—Current Chapter Title." For example, "July 1, 2015, Mary's Marvelous Transformation— Introduction." (You will write the same heading at the beginning of each new chapter, for example, "July 1, 2015, Mary's Marvelous Transformation—Chapter 1.")

2. Take ten minutes (set a timer if you can) to purge your mind and soul of your thoughts and feelings about your condition. It can be in the style of stream-of-consciousness writing or a simple bulleted list, whichever suits you best. Describe or make a list of the things you currently think, feel, and believe about

your health, your life, your limitations and successes, and your wants and desires. These instructions are purposely vague and open-ended. There is nothing too small, silly, strange, intense, or superficial to write down.

3. After ten minutes, stop writing, take a deep breath, and allow yourself a moment to process what you wrote. Read it over and notice if any points, either as you wrote them or now while you are reviewing them, cause a physical reaction within you. Do you notice any physical pain or sensations like heart racing, body tingling, stabbing, or lifting? Do you feel a knot in your stomach? Did you tear up at any point? Did you laugh? Feel embarrassed? Take note of the items that resonate most powerfully for you and circle them (it could be single words, phrases, or a particular paragraph). Any physical or emotional reaction is an indicator that you've put your finger on a raw element that you are ready to address and heal. The items you circled are the most potentially transformative issues in your life. Congratulations for having identified them.

4. Next, turn the page and draw a vertical line down the middle of it. Look at your circled items and find the ones that express something negative (it may be all of them, and that is perfectly okay). For each negative feeling or thought you circled, formulate a declarative sentence that expresses the issue. For example, you may have circled the phrase, "I don't think this next treatment will solve anything and I'm close to giving up hope." You would translate this into the simple sentence: "I feel hopeless." If you

wrote a bulleted list and one of the words was "sad," turn it into the declarative statement, "I feel sad" or "I am always sad." Write these negative sentences to the left of your vertical line.

5. When you have a statement for each of the negative circled items in the left column (perhaps it's one or two, or maybe you've written two dozen—however it unfolds is exactly how it's meant to be), go back to the top and consider the first statement. Think about what the exact opposite of that negative statement would be, and write it down in the right-hand column. For example, if you wrote "I feel hopeless," the positive opposite could be "I have hope." If you wrote "I'm afraid," write "I'm brave." If you wrote "Life sucks," the opposite could be "Life is beautiful." If you wrote "I'm tired and can't take this anymore," the counter might be "I am full of energy and can handle anything that comes my way." Make sure you complete the whole list and come up with a positive counter statement to each of your negative sentences. You may notice as you write the opposite to each negative thought or feeling that a part of you can't help but agree with the positive statement. You really do have hope. Life really is beautiful. You truly are strong. If you don't feel the truth in any of the opposite assertions right now, that's okay, too. Transformations don't have to happen overnight. Simply allow your mind to absorb the positive opposites to what you originally expressed, and trust that your subconscious is listening. For now, just allow these positive truths to live on the pages of your journal. We will come back to them later.

Chapter One

Diagnosis:
Shifting Realities

Take Stock of Where You Are Now

In your journal, write briefly in response to the following questions.
One or two sentences for each will suffice.

1. How easy, or difficult, was your diagnosis process?

2. For how long did you experience symptoms before you started getting answers?

3. What was it like for you when you were waiting for a diagnosis? What thoughts did you have?

4. How did you feel when you finally had a diagnosis?

5. How did your world change?

6. How do you feel, now, when you think back to that time?

The Wonderful Pieces of Divinity
I Have Found

Humor is your friend.

.

Appreciate the little things.

.

Sometimes your mood comes down to a choice.
Do you want to be happy or sad today?

.

People help you as a way of showing love
when they feel helpless against your disease.

.

You may not control your disease,
but you control how you think and feel about it.
Therefore, you control your experience.

My road to autoimmunity is probably similar to yours or your loved one's. I had countless environmental sensitivities as a child. Temperature changes, humidity, and barometric pressure changes affected me, as did chemicals in shampoos and detergents—even fabrics. I had respiratory infections, strange rashes, and excruciating muscle pains. I also found myself to be fairly clumsy. Aside from all those pesky inconveniences, I was a normal, physically active, energetic kid, full of life and zest for adventure. Does this sound familiar?

We had traces of autoimmunity in our family—a bit of arthritis and psoriasis—and there were various forms of cancer, but nothing so unusual as to indicate we were at higher risk than the general population.

In my second year of college, I contracted mononucleosis. Prior to being diagnosed, I was put on antibiotics, which triggered an allergic reaction that caused an all-over-body-rash the likes of which few have ever seen.

This event, the raging mononucleosis, was the final catalyst that took me from having an overly sensitive body, which made me a *candidate* for problems, to someone whose immune system went undeniably haywire. My immune system forgot what it was supposed to do (protect the body from germs) and went on the offensive (attacking itself) instead.

Over the next eight years, I saw numerous doctors and had many tests and various diagnoses before we settled on what they believed was the correct single diagnosis: juvenile-onset dermatomyositis.

The snippets of information I received from the pre-diagnosis doctors were big words like lupus, multiple sclerosis, muscular dystrophy, and cancer. During that time I was alternately called delusional, a hypochondriac, a liar, and an insomniac, or they said that I had *only* fibromyalgia—just to name a few. In the years since, and as understanding has increased, the qualifier "only" has been removed from any mention of fibromyalgia.

Have They Given You Meds, Meds, and More Meds?

I felt like a guinea pig being put on medicine after medicine to treat, or rather diagnose, the symptoms of the disease. More meds were needed to treat the side effects of the initial meds, and still more to treat the side effects of those. I saw some wonderful doctors as well as many others who clearly should have chosen a different career.

As a child I knew a woman who died in childbirth from undiagnosed lupus, so I was scared out of my wits. The prognosis for someone with lupus wasn't good, yet I didn't feel like I was supposed to die. The doctor my parents took me to said he wasn't sure *what* was wrong with me. Possibly it could resolve itself and turn out to be minor. In any case, he wasn't going to diagnose me because of my age.

This was hard to digest. Was it that I wasn't ill enough to warrant a diagnosis? Or that it wasn't clear? Was it just his way of saying he didn't know? My stepdad would helpfully point out that the lack of definitive answers from doctors is the reason they are said to be practicing medicine.

I spent much of my twenties feeling like my head was halfway in the guillotine, waiting to be shoved all the way in so that someone could deliver my death sentence and lower the big boom.

In teaching hospitals I was poked and prodded by thirty-plus medical students who said things like, "Wow, that rash is really cool!" Never mind I was a human being, in pain, scared out of my mind, and wishing I could be anywhere but here, and have clear skin without a painful, oozing rash (a major indicator that whatever my ailment, it was in full form). Could it be fatal?

Thanks so much, dear, young medical student, for telling me how cool this rash is.

Instead of saying that I just smiled and listened—and then cried when I got to my car. If you've ever visited a teaching hospital, you may have experienced the same sort of insensitivity. Did you find it hard to remember that they were young and immature and didn't mean to dehumanize you? I did.

I had full-fledged doctors who, by the way, didn't have my disease, tell me to buck up and get over it; it wasn't *that* painful. How could they possibly know? They implied I was exaggerating when I said I couldn't walk up a flight of stairs; maybe it was all depression and that I should stop looking for an excuse to be sad; or there were people much sicker than me and that I should be grateful I didn't have a terminal disease like the person they saw in the last room.

Why did people who didn't live my life feel they had the right to tell me how I should or should not be feeling, or how much pain I should or should not be experiencing? I wondered why these people had gone to medical school if they already thought they knew everything.

Raw Emotions During Your "Limbo" Time

If you remember the emotions you felt while going through your "limbo" time—the time before diagnosis—know you are in good company. Many, perhaps most, autoimmunity patients go through years of misdiagnoses before getting the correct one. It's upsetting, frustrating, and scary.

What a relief it was to finally have an actual diagnosis. I wondered if it meant I was glad to be sick, but I realized it wasn't. I was just happy to have answers so I could finally move forward.

Before and immediately after the diagnosis, my life changed dramatically. My education and jobs were affected. I was fortunate to have some understanding bosses who allowed me flexible hours, or coworkers who picked up the slack when I was exhausted. When I knew I was getting close to using up sick days, I would look for a new job; this usually happened around the six-month mark. Repeatedly.

My resume from the first couple of years after college looks a bit like hopscotch. I had five different jobs between January 1998 and April 2000, and it wasn't my work ethic. I outwardly blamed it on needing to find myself, but my dark secret was that I was always one step ahead of being fired for absences. If it wasn't one aspect of my illness, it was another; I started thinking I was making it up myself. I was twenty-two years old and barely able to function.

The Effect on Your Family

People talk about how chronic illness tears families apart; this can certainly be true. It is stressful to feel sick all the time, and I know how stressful it is for my husband, Scott. Even on days when he has a project due at work, I have to call him, crying about how badly I hurt and how I cannot get out of bed to make lunch for our daughter. He comes home to care for us, despite the inconvenience.

Or the days when there isn't anything wrong except I am so fatigued that lifting my arm feels like a full workout. Scott steps in without fail and takes over everything in the house. Consider the heap of medical bills we incur every year that he somehow finds a way to manage. Even though we have insurance, with deductibles—which I've used up by January each year for the past eight years—we are never without an overwhelming amount of medical debt.

There are times I'm sure he would just like to come home from a long day at work to a normal stay-at-home wife and mother, a clean house, and a ready meal. I bet he wishes he didn't have to do the dishes because my hands are too weak and sensitive to the hot water; carry the laundry up the stairs or vacuum because I am not strong enough; haul out the trash; or perform any of the dozens of chores I am unable to do even on my best day.

I watched Scott go through our two miscarriages. Yes, they were likely due to autoimmunity, as the body tries to eliminate the fetus in utero, attacking it and cutting off its flow of nutrients because the body sees it as a threat to my health. It's hard enough for me to go through a miscarriage, but watching my love lose his children at the same time, too, and knowing it is because my body failed to carry them—there aren't words for the pain and the guilt I feel.

Sage, our little girl, is a miracle. She is here by the grace of God, my sheer will, a dedicated high-risk prenatal doctor, my acupuncturist, and some immunosuppressant drugs. Together we coaxed and cajoled my body into holding on to her and bringing her into the world—safely.

Loved ones of people with chronic diseases take on a lot more than they bargained for. My husband knew I was sick, and he chose to love me anyway. I didn't sugarcoat it when we were dating. I didn't yet have a specific diagnosis, but I told him what life might be like with me. He chose to be with me anyway. He agreed to be there for me when I couldn't take care of myself, and he lives up to that promise every day. It is not easy for me to watch him make those sacrifices.

Expect Everything to Be Affected

Even prior to diagnosis, autoimmunity played a key role in my relationships. It affects everything, from your everyday decisions to your emotional stability and trust in yourself and your partner— even your sexual relationships. A former partner would carry me up the stairs of my apartment because my hips and legs were so weak I would have had to crawl if I'd been alone. You don't know vulnerability until you become that dependent on another human being. At the same time, you are also gifted with the beautiful opportunity to feel loved and cared for on a different level.

It can be hardest for your parents. I hear my dad cry on the phone at any health news, both good and bad. I watch my mom wrestle with worry over every little test and appointment. As a mom myself, I know how helpless my parents must feel watching their "baby" in pain and not being able to fix it. They, too, have done everything they can to help, sometimes to the point of smothering me.

Friends have played a huge part in enabling me to continue living in a way that resembles normalcy. Yet they are the first to suffer the consequences of broken promises and broken dates when I cannot go through with plans.

Autoimmunity doesn't just happen to the person who's blood tests, magnetic resonance imaging (MRI) tests, electromyograms (EMGs), and biopsies turn up positive for the disease. Autoimmunity also happens to families, friends, and coworkers. With this book, I want to honor not just "us" who are the patients but "us" who are the people—the community—who help us patients keep going.

I have often wondered whether death would be a merciful escape and hear this from other patients as well. Perhaps you have even been there yourself. But I promise those moments are fleeting. People around me have helped me decide to keep going in the darkest of hours, and I hope this sharing of my experiences will help you decide you can keep going as well.

What "You Create Your Own Reality" Means

As hinted at in Neale's quote, the idea that we create our own reality has been misinterpreted to imply that if only we are strong enough, we can cast disease from our bodies through thought alone. Anyone who has suffered from autoimmune disease knows the callous ignorance underlying such claims. What creating your own reality really means is to cultivate your ability to create and take responsibility for the mental environment within which you operate, thereby ending your emotional suffering so that you can face your disease head-on—with acceptance, strength, and laughter. It is not meant to cause you guilt or shame.

When I stop feeling angry about my disease, my whole world changes. It doesn't mean that I am physically healed or that the disease is gone, it means that I find ways to appreciate my life as it is. Sometimes I have to put "mind over matter" and be happy with my life, even if my body isn't performing the way I wish it would.

There are ways in which my life has been enhanced because of my disease: I have become someone I like much better than the person I would have been if I hadn't been so challenged; and I have established a deeper connection to divinity because of my experiences with this illness. Now I understand that having a shifted reality (diagnosis) doesn't have to equate to suffering (a decrease in the quality of my inner landscape); I can choose happiness.

This book won't heal your disease. But it will help you heal your ideas about the disease and find ways to love your body and your life, sometimes despite the disease, sometimes in celebration of it—and often through humorous reflection on it.

Creative Tips for Empowering Yourself

- While the diagnosis stage is scary, remember you are still the same person you were before. Whether your diagnosis is recent or not, remember you are not your disease; you merely have it. Say, "I am a person with these symptoms," or "My body is healthy, whole, and happy!" By doing so, you maintain your own identity and remember that your life is not controlled by illness.

- Find one thing to laugh about today.

- Pick one thing you did today, however small, that you couldn't do yesterday and say "thank you" to your body.

- Replace anger with acceptance and gratitude. Say, "It's okay that I can't do everything I want to do; I will celebrate the things I *can* do."

- Repeat after me: "I can be happy no matter what is happening to my body because I am a beautiful, wonderful being, and I am alive!"

Caregiver Tips

- For any parent, spouse, significant other, or close friend, the beginning stages of diagnosis are scary—know you are an important part of your loved one's journey.

- To be supportive of your loved one, listen to him or her, accompany him or her, be understanding, and realize you don't have to "solve" everything to help.

- Just being there is often enough.

Create Your Own Marvelous Transformation

Take your journal and spend a few minutes reflecting on what you've just read. Let the following questions guide you in processing your own truth and emotionally charged experiences you may have been reminded of through reading my story. Thinking and writing about these ideas and any positive insights you have gained from this chapter will help internalize and solidify your own transformation:

1. What situation or example in this chapter resonated most with you?

2. When faced with similar situations, how do you feel, act, or think?

3. What would you most like to remember from this chapter?

4. What can you do going forward to view your diagnosis in a more positive light?

5. How do you feel, now, when you think back to the time of your diagnosis?

6. With your new perspective, how will you deal with feelings of unfairness from now on?

7. Look back at the notes you made before you read this chapter. Have your thoughts changed after reading the chapter? If so, how? What realizations are you most grateful for?

Chapter Two

Pigtails and Knobby Knees: Learning to Overcome

Take Stock of Where You Are Now

Transformations often begin with a radical decision. Answer the following questions about life-changing decisions in your journal.

1. Name a time when you changed a habit or trait that no longer served you.

2. What did you do to change the habit or trait?

3. How did you feel about the decision?

4. What was the experience of change like (easy or difficult) once you made the decision?

5. What parts of your life have been altered due to your health?

6. Describe any tough decisions you've had to make to change your chosen path. How do you feel about those decisions?

7. If there were another area in your life in which you could make a powerful, path-altering decision, what would it be? How do you feel when you think about making that change?

The Wonderful Pieces of Divinity
I Have Found

You are stronger than you know,
even if you have to dig deep to find it.

.

You can do anything you put your mind to.

.

Be grateful for the life you have.

.

Having autoimmunity helps you slow down.
This is a good thing.

.

Money isn't everything.

.

Your planned career may not have been your life purpose;
find your path by listening to life as it presents itself.

I was that awkward, shy, creative, pigtailed girl with her nose stuck in a book on the playground. The middle of three kids, I was quiet and didn't really understand other people's jokes. I tried to be nice to everyone and while I wanted to have a lot of friends, whenever I found myself in a crowd of kids I just wanted to be left alone. The only place I felt truly comfortable was with my family. This shyness would play a huge role in my ability to manage my health later in life.

Mom stayed home and chauffeured the three of us around, as mothers do, until she became a teacher when I was in third grade. She liked to sew a lot. She enjoyed decorating and sewing, making some of our clothes and all of our Halloween costumes. We could dress up as whomever and whatever we wanted: a mermaid, a bride, a pumpkin, you name it. Today I love making my own daughter's Halloween costumes, thanks to those wonderful memories.

Dad worked in construction and would smell of sweat and bitter asphalt when he came home. We had a few dogs over the years and an above-ground swimming pool with a wooden deck that my dad and some neighbors built with their own hands and, likely, a few beers. Dad always had some home improvement project going on, including once cutting a hole in the ceiling to relocate our bedrooms in the attic; five years later we finally moved into those new rooms. My parents still can't agree on whose ideas the home construction projects were, but suffice it to say our life was a constant adventure.

Mom and Dad worked hard to give us what we needed, and we had a fun-filled childhood. We played games, rode bikes, and had movie nights. We knew we were loved; we never doubted that, ever.

My grandparents lived one block from my school, so I saw my grandma every day. She was only four-foot-ten but had a personality that filled the entire room. Sometimes I pretended to be sick just to get a day alone with Grandma without my siblings. I would lie on her sofa and watch her "soapies" with her. Since I was sick, I wasn't allowed to get up and play; of course, she knew if I was faking, but I don't think she cared. She would make me grilled cheese or egg salad sandwiches, or whatever my current favorite food was. When Mom came home those evenings, Grandma would be the one who was hoarse because I had talked her ear off all day, forcing her to keep up.

I was an overachiever and harder on myself than my parents were when I didn't do as well as I wanted in school. Books were my best friends. I would sneak off to the bathroom to read, rather than help clean on Saturdays. On road trips I would read an entire book in a couple of hours. We had to bring a bag of books for me alone if it was a long drive.

I remained painfully shy all through high school, and though I had a core group of close friends, I never did become the social butterfly my family believed I was.

One day our family welcomed my sweet nephew, Rickey. Since he lived with us, I had the pleasure of seeing him every day, and he brought an unrivaled light and joy to my life. His existence convinced me I wanted to be a mom someday. He fit into our family like a glove and became one of the few people with whom I was free to be myself. His little mop-top of black hair and his infectious laugh continue to steal the show, and our hearts, to this day.

It Could Be Your Most Powerful Tool

When I went away to college I made my first mind-over-matter decision. If I continued being shy and quiet, I would be back home within weeks because of my loneliness, so I decided that was not an option. I had scholarships and big plans. Having emerged from the shadows of my siblings—my unpredictable older sister and my gregarious, sporty younger brother—there was no going back. As my parents pulled away after delivering me to the campus, I reinvented myself and shed my shyness like a second skin.

I acted like the person I'd always wanted to be: outgoing, fun, and unafraid. In the first few days on campus, I walked up to three people and introduced myself; this was something I would never have done before (and I'm glad I did because all three are my soul companions to this day).

When I tell people how shy I still feel inside, especially those I didn't know until college, their response is always the same: "There's no way you are shy. You have to be making that up."

Only my closest friends knew the truth. Every new interaction was painful for me, and I doubted each word that came out of my own mouth. Replaying every conversation, I would second-guess even my body movements. While I wasn't always received the way

I wanted to be, I did learn I was a lot stronger than I had thought. I realized self-perception was the only reality that mattered. I proved to myself that if I set my mind to something I could accomplish it, to the point of creating a whole new version of myself.

The recognition that I can control my thoughts about myself and my circumstances has become a powerful tool in dealing with my disease and with life in general. I share this because I believe it can be a powerful tool for you as well—perhaps the most powerful.

I met and married the love of my life, Scott, after a few false starts and missteps in my early adulthood. Those experiences helped me become who I am and prepared me for the beautiful life I have with him. Despite the youthful emotional pain of those early encounters, I am grateful for them.

Scott is patient, kind, and giving. He may get annoyed with my physical limitations, but he has never—not once in our marriage— let it show. Dermatomyositis taught me how to slow down and enjoy the important, tender things in life; my marriage is definitely part of that gift.

At some point along the way I embarked on a spiritual quest. I'd been raised to go to church but had never been satisfied with it. As a young child I questioned things I felt were inconsistent. When I first read Neale's *Conversations with God* and heard its nonjudgmental messages of oneness and love, I knew it was exactly what I'd believed all along but had been afraid to say. I embraced my inner knowing and haven't looked back since.

Stand Ready to Make Daring Decisions

After graduating from law school and passing the bar exam, I made a daring decision. With an enormous amount of debt and three-and-a-half years of school behind me, I decided that being a lawyer didn't suit me after all. Too bad I couldn't figure that out without all the schooling and the debt, but I am stubborn—just ask Dad. I had to see it all, digest it, and learn it for myself.

It was not an easy decision to make. Remember that supportive husband I was talking about earlier? You should have seen his face when I said, "Um, Honey, I'm not sure being a lawyer is really for me." But as we examined it together, my decision made sense for us. First, we looked at my day-to-day health. I'd finally been diagnosed while in law school, and I was getting worse, so our thoughts had to change on some things.

Chronic migraines, all-over pain, vibrational feelings from fibromyalgia, down days due to dermatomyositis (any one of which can put me in bed for days on end), and my previous job history—it all added up to the inevitable conclusion that I'd have trouble holding down a job. Stress and fatigue play a major role in autoimmune disease, and I'd be hard-pressed to find a position with a legal firm that was limited to forty hours a week, if I could even put in that much time.

Then there was the fact that Scott is also an attorney who works many overtime hours—and we were having a child. We didn't want a nanny to raise her, so it wasn't feasible for both of us to work full-time—especially if it was going to be detrimental to my health. Nagging at the back of my mind, whether I admitted it or not, was also the question of how many years I had left. After all, I have a chronic, degenerative, and possibly fatal disease. Would working hasten that? Would it make me miss more of my daughter's life?

If that wasn't enough, my ideas about the world had changed over the years at law school, and I realized if I was going to practice full-time, I would prefer it to be with a human rights, nonprofit organization. This might have to be in another city or another country, and would likely not pay enough for day care, much less help with the student loan payments.

The best solution appeared to be to start a solo practice doing wills from home and seeing how that would go. We tried that for a while, but though I did a good job on the work I took in, my heart wasn't in it. My health interfered even with the few legal engagements I had outside the house. I was also required to take continuing legal education (CLE) courses, and the extra load inevitably led to extreme fatigue and migraines.

After just a few years I decided to let my law license lapse rather than continuing to waste money and time keeping it active for pride's sake. The relief was immense. It was one of those moments in which I got to decide the course of my life, instead of allowing past decisions to dictate my current happiness.

Without the stress of having to complete the CLEs and paying for my license, and with no more guilt about not actively looking for clients, I was breathing easier. And, just like the skin of shyness, I shed my life as a lawyer.

Today I serve on the board of directors of The Myositis Support and Understanding Association (MSU), write my *With My Child* series of children's books, blog on health and parenting, write articles and essays for nontraditional spirituality publications, and I coauthored the book *Conversations with God for Parents* with Neale Donald Walsch and Laurie Lankins Farley. It is much easier to deal with my disease when I can work at my own pace and on my own schedule. I can sleep or take breaks to get refreshed and recharged as needed.

A Great Secret: Accept Changes Happily

Changes come in all shapes and sizes. What kind of changes have you had to make in order to accommodate your limitations? Many people continue to work but find less strenuous and stressful jobs. Thankfully, those who are unable to work at all are often able to utilize governmental assistance for income.

I am fortunate to be able to stay home and my husband has been able to support us along with what little supplementary income I provide. We have made sacrifices and have our share of financial stresses—student loans and medical bills don't pay themselves. I haven't always been a financial help, and often I've been more of a drain on our finances. However, I make my contribution to our family in other ways.

My most important contribution is that I homeschool our daughter. There are myriad reasons why I do so, including the quality of her education, our knowledge about how she learns best, our wish to be the strongest influence in her life for a while longer, and our desire to help her become a creative thinker. We also have to consider that it shields me from the germs she would bring home from school if she were there on a daily basis. I've been on immunosuppressant drugs the majority of the last twenty years, and, ironically, these drugs make you more susceptible to germs. I joke that a fly can sneeze a few rooms away and I will get a cold—an exaggeration, but it illustrates how vulnerable, in fact, I am.

Learn to Be Cautious

Prior to play dates, birthday parties, and dinners, my friends must get frustrated with my calls asking if anyone is sick. They may think I'm paranoid. Nevertheless, the level of caution I've adopted is necessary to protect myself. It's hard to cancel plans at the last minute because someone in the other family is sick, but the repercussions of *not* canceling are harder on my family than most people can even imagine. I can only hope for people's understanding.

Not only am I more susceptible to germs, but I've learned the cold it takes the average person a short time to get over can be a big deal for me. I can't count the number of times I've seen my husband, nephew, or daughter sniffle for two days, only to find myself in bed for two weeks with a full-blown flare-up of my disease.

We are cautious when going out in public during cold and flu season. Hand sanitizer is never far from my reach. Minimizing my exposure by minimizing my daughter's exposure through homeschooling her has helped enormously. But there are other, positive, reasons as well why homeschooling has become one of the greatest joys in my life. I get to watch my daughter learn, witness her brain developing, and see new things swirl around and finally click when she gets them.

This is one of the gifts of autoimmunity. I would not have considered homeschooling had I been healthy and ready to take on the legal world. I would have sent my child off to school without thinking of germs, without stopping to make a conscious choice about what might work better for our family, and without considering being a stay-at-home mom in the long-term. I would have remained on a traditional career path and tried to balance it all, in the end missing precious time with my sweet baby. For all of the wonderful moments with my lovely daughter—my little miracle—I say, "Thank you, Dermatomyositis!"

Creative Tips for Empowering Yourself

- Listen to life as it occurs; learn to resonate with your true needs. Starting with small circumstances, begin really listening to your heart and intuition. You can start by asking yourself a simple question: "Does this situation feel right, or am I doing it because of what others expect of me?" Making conscious choices gives you back a sense of power and control when you feel you lack the same over your body. You know what is best for your health if you will just take the time to listen. As you get more practiced at the little daily tasks, you can examine your bigger life decisions. Sometimes our planned course of action is not what works best for us.

- Give yourself permission and take the time to enjoy the view along the way.

- Get out your journal and think back to a time when you exhibited more inner strength than you knew you had. Remember where you found it and how it felt to use it. Write it down. Describe how your true self is showing up for you. Whenever you are feeling weak or defeated, reread this entry and remind yourself of who you really are inside. Add other great strength moments to the list as they arise, and you'll maintain a living document that allows you to see how amazing you are.

- Repeat after me: "I can take control of my own destiny."

Caregiver Tips

- Know that your loved one may have to make decisions that might seem "outside the plan" at first, but those decisions will greatly enhance health, and, therefore, daily life.

- Be prepared for a loss of income. Spending adjustments will need to be made in order to support the necessary health-related decisions.

- Assure your loved one that he or she need not feel guilty about any of this, and allow yourself to know that dealing with chronic disease is difficult enough, without feeling terrible about the effects it is having on your family.

- Understand that just as your loved one's life and physical reality has changed with autoimmunity, your life will change as well.

- Be patient with your loved one; he or she is more frustrated with the changes than you are. With the loss of independence, dignity suffers.

- You may be asked to take on more housework and more physical and emotional responsibility in your relationship. Are you ready and willing to do so? Just as your loved one might wish to seek professional support in dealing with the changes, it could be beneficial for you as well.

- You may offer support through back rubs and foot and arm massage, which can be extremely comforting to your loved one.

Create Your Own Marvelous Transformation

Grab your journal and spend a few minutes contemplating what you just read. Use the following questions to guide you.

1. What situation or example resonated most with you in this chapter?

2. When faced with a similar situation, how do you feel, act, or think?

3. What would you most like to remember from this chapter?

Now we're going to take this to the next level. You are going to make your own mind-over-matter decision, right here, right now. Follow these steps, and don't skip any of the hard parts. The more thought, time, care, and attention you invest, the greater your rewards will be.

1. Set aside an hour of uninterrupted time, where you can focus on yourself and don't need to worry about any family, social, or work obligations. If you can do that right now, wonderful; if not, go ahead and mark a date in your calendar. Make any necessary arrangements (childcare, etc.), or simply let your partner and family members know that you will be unavailable at this specified time. Do not try to skip this step or squeeze it into a five minute window.

2. Now that you have an hour scheduled for yourself, find a quiet place where you can be undisturbed for the duration of that time. Do whatever form of mental and spiritual preparation works best for you, and make sure you are in a centered, calm, and relaxed frame of mind. Now meditate, pray, or otherwise think deeply about the life you want to lead. Your ideal life. Let there be no boundaries, no limitations. No dream is too big. Allow your subconscious to put it all out there for your conscious self to see. Spend at least ten minutes thinking about the question. What is your ideal life? How do you feel there? What do you find yourself doing? Who are the people around you? What is the place or space around you? What are the activities you're doing and the sights

and sounds you're absorbing? What does it feel like to be this happy? Let it resonate with you. Feel it in your body, in your gut, and in your cells. Let the sensations of living your ideal life wash over you.

3. When you're done glimpsing into your ideal life, "download" as much of what you've just seen onto paper. Spend a good twenty minutes on this. Write notes, draw pictures, or write a poem— anything to capture what your dream life looks and feels like. Take special note of anything related to the senses. What clothes were you wearing? What colors surrounded you? What was the weather like? What aromas and tastes made you happy? The activities you were enjoying: what did they feel like to the touch? Focusing on these elements helps you side-step the logical and limiting part of your mind, giving you greater and more unmediated access to the details of your ideal life.

4. When you feel you've gotten the essence of your dream life captured on paper, sit back and take it all in. Which aspect of the dream—what real-life goal—can you identify that, if you pursued it successfully, would bring about the *most* elements of your ideal life with the *least* amount of time and effort? Allow another ten minutes for this thinking process. Don't get overwhelmed with everything you think you could or should be doing; all you have to do right now is find and pick the one thing—that one activity, task, accomplishment, or change—that would get you closest to your dream in the shortest amount of time. For example, let's say your dream is to own your own restaurant in an exotic location,

where you spend your days cooking up exquisite five-star gala dinners for a glamorous clientele. For right now, your task would not be to find and apply for a program at a culinary school. Rather, you might simply make a commitment to cooking a festive meal for your family once a week and, perhaps, to challenge yourself to learn something new by using a new cookbook, looking up a new recipe online, or finding a magazine with five-star culinary ideas. The point is to hone in on what you can do in your life right now, realistically and attainably, to bring you closer to your ideal life. If you had more than one dream (and most of us do), focus on the one that makes you feel most alive. Then identify and formulate a realistic goal toward making that dream (the activities and experiences associated with the happiness you feel in the dream) a reality.

5. Now, think about and list the steps it will take to accomplish your goal. This should take another ten minutes or so. If you pictured yourself running a marathon, outline what you might have to do to get there, such as taking medicines as prescribed, attending aquatic therapy to start building muscles, doing yoga, walking around the block, walking to the store, joining a gym and walking a track, completing a 5K, or completing a half marathon. If you saw yourself in a specific career, write down the steps to achieve it, such as going to school, getting an internship, or making connections in the field.

6. Finally, for the remaining ten minutes, break down the steps you've listed and incorporate them into your daily life and

schedule. Set dates, schedule appointments, make a to do list for today, tomorrow, next week, next month, and so on. Consider how this goal and your new commitment to it will affect your loved ones and your other existing commitments, and think of ways in which you can prepare and accommodate them. At the end of the hour, ground yourself again in whichever way works best for you, and close your mind-over-matter session with an expression of appreciation. Thank the universe for the inspiration and guidance you've received, and express your gratitude for all it is doing for you (whether fully realized or yet in process). You could say, "I am grateful for my health" (no matter what level of it you have right now), "I am grateful for my family," "I love my home," "I am excited to experience working toward my new goal," "I look forward to that trip I am going to take" (even if it isn't planned yet), or "Thank you (God, Universe, my self, etc.) for the financial security I am experiencing."

I've never run a marathon, but a few years ago I was able to work up to running six miles, from having trouble walking to the end of my driveway. It is one of the most fulfilling physical successes I've experienced in my life. It was short lived, but I did it! I wanted to run a marathon and was about to commit to training for it when one of my flares hit. I didn't run the marathon, or even continue running six miles, but the accomplishments I had along the way made up for it.

Ponder these words: "I have no attachment to results." For me this means that I set goals, work at them, and appreciate the journey, knowing that sometimes the end result may look different from what I have envisioned. I have come to know that this is okay. I haven't failed if I don't reach my planned outcome because each step along the way has its own reward, and I often end up in places or situations I have never imagined.

1. Take your journal and jot down your thoughts on how you can apply "I have no attachment to the results" in your life. Some part of your life is crying out for you to embrace this idea. Which is it? What will it relieve within you when you start believing it?

2. Finally, look back at the notes you made before you read this chapter. How have your thoughts and feelings changed since then?

Chapter Three

I Am So Scared: Why Dr. Smartphone Is Not Your Friend

Take Stock of Where You Are Now

Take a few minutes and reflect on the following questions, writing down your thoughts in response to each in brief sentences.

1. To what extent do you rely on the internet to answer your medical questions?

2. Why? Write down two to three specific instances when you thought it was a good idea to research online.

3. What was it that you expected to find?

4. Was it worth it? How did the experience turn out in each case?

5. What reaction did you have to what you found?

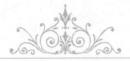

The Wonderful Pieces of Divinity
I Have Found

Trust your instincts—not Dr. Smartphone.

·

When you get scared, remember to feel it and
let it pass through you, instead of holding on to it.

·

Embrace patience; be okay with not knowing
everything right now.

·

Celebrate the small victories!

When any one of us feel out of control or unclear about a physical condition, what do we do? We grab our smartphones or computers and search the Internet. Google, WebMD, Yahoo, and Wikipedia may seem helpful, but sometimes they are not such a good idea. One time while researching online, I convinced myself I had every disease and disorder known to mankind. Well, almost.

The feeling of loss of control is devastating when you develop health issues. For many years my body felt like it was being smashed down, strung up, lit on fire, pulled out, ground between two metal vices, and generally beaten down—on a daily basis. From the time my symptoms started, I had dreams that my teeth were crumbling and falling out—a sign of feeling out of control. Did I ever! Only my closest family and friends could understand a fraction of what I was experiencing, but even their tolerance, understanding, and patience wore thin at times.

I don't always feel out of control; I have moments when I feel great, when I know I am beating the odds, and when I know that science and medicine have come a long way. I remember that I am fortunate to have the juvenile form of the disease because it has a lower mortality rate.

Scott and I came to know a wonderful woman who was diagnosed with adult onset dermatomyositis. She struggled and fought a courageous battle but died within a couple of years. Her death affected me profoundly. All the resolve that I had built up, all the hope that I was going to be okay, that I could beat and conquer this condition, melted in an instant. At the same time I mourned and wept for my friend and her family, I wept for myself. All my fears and the feelings of loss of control returned.

One Thing You May *Not* Want to Do

Internet diagnosing is a problem for me because the symptoms are written so vaguely that anyone can fit the description. The online examples are usually the worst-case scenarios that can scare the heck out of you. My determination to become my own doctor, after the medical doctors couldn't tell me what was wrong, failed me miserably. I became a hypochondriac—in a cruel twist of irony, just what some of those doctors had said I was.

Every new symptom made me think I was going to die of a new manifestation of my disease. Every article I read had me convinced that I would:

- be in a wheelchair by the time I was thirty,

- never have a child,

- balloon to 500 pounds from the prednisone,

- become psychotic from the medications, and

- die within five years.

And this list is by no means complete.

Every time my disease progressed, it sent me back to the Internet for more information to mislead me. Eventually I understood that my independent research was not helping me re-establish control over my life. It was causing me to slip further down into the hole of fear and uncertainty.

Can You Make a Promise with Me?

How do you deal with the need to control everything? I remind myself that I can only control my own thoughts and feelings. I breathe deeply—a lot. I practice acceptance and gratitude. I do yoga (more about that later).

I made a commitment to myself that I wouldn't rely on Dr. Smartphone for diagnoses and treatment of my disease. I asked my husband and other loved ones around me to assist in my quest to avoid self-diagnosis in case I fall off the wagon. When a new symptom arises, they remind me.

Even when I don't agree, I will allow the professionals to do their jobs, and then I will discuss (or argue) the things I don't agree on with them. When a new problem crops up, it's not time to do more research but time to reach for the phone and make an appointment with my doctor.

Can you make that commitment with me?

Creative Tips for Empowering Yourself

- Online information is usually written very broadly. It can be written by anyone with no evidence to back it up. Take anything you read online with a grain of salt. There are *some* organizations that endeavor to give good, reliable information. They are listed in the Appendix for your reference.

- When you feel the need for control and the desire to research, take a deep breath. Remember the only things you can control are your emotions and your responses to them. Practicing patience and restraint is far easier than dealing with anxiety from misinformation.

- When in doubt, go see your healthcare professional.

- If you feel you are in immediate danger, it is safer to seek emergency medical attention than to attempt self-diagnosis on the Internet.

- Make a commitment now to breathe and tell yourself, "I am a unique individual with specific needs. Online information is too vague to help me; I deserve better than that."

Caregiver Tips

- Medical terms for physical conditions can be scary. Don't tell your loved one "not to be afraid." Rather, give assurance that you understand his or her fear, that it is perfectly normal, and that you will help deal with the fear. Your loved one's anxiety can be reduced by simply allowing him or her to talk about it; even if it means listening to what you have already heard many times. Repetition can be helpful to the patient, providing a peaceful and supportive feeling that he or she is at least being heard.

- Feeling out of control adds to fear and stress. Consider helping your loved one find some level of control over circumstances.

- Encourage your loved one to consult with a doctor if conditions change or become worrisome and to resist the urge to look up symptoms online.

Create Your Own Marvelous Transformation

Take some time now to integrate what you've read in this chapter, using the following questions to guide you.

1. What situation or example resonated most with you in this chapter?

2. When faced with a similar situation, how do you feel, act, or think?

3. What would you most like to remember from this chapter?

4. Now, flip to a new page in your journal or notepad. Down the left-hand side of the page, make a list of all the symptoms you know that can occur with your disease. Include your own existing symptoms as well as ones you know of and are worried about but haven't experienced yourself. When you're done with the list, go back to the top. Next to each symptom you have actually experienced, place a checkmark. For the ones you haven't experienced, write a number between one and ten to indicate how much each worries you, where one means "I'm not scared at all," and ten means "I am petrified!" Next to any symptom for which you rated your fear at a five or higher, write a positive affirmation of health. Try not to use any negative wording (such as "I am glad I don't have . . .") but use positive language instead. For example, if the symptom is "calcinosis," write: "I am grateful that my skin, muscles, and tendons are clear with smooth transitions and free from deposits."

5. Now create a new habit for yourself. Whenever you have a negative thought or fear, allow it to come fully into existence and into consciousness. Acknowledge its presence, allowing your body, mind, and soul to express the fear and then—transform

it! The point is not to ignore your fears but not to dwell on them either. Acknowledge the thoughts, and then change them. You have the power and the ability to change the thought, the very instant you have it, into a positive affirmation of gratitude. For example, if your thought is, "My body is not working," acknowledge it, sit with it, and don't resist it. Affirm it. Then, let it communicate what it wants to communicate, and simply transform it by saying, for instance, "My body works very hard to be healthy, and I am grateful." Or the thought, "This is so painful, I wish it would stop!" can be transformed into "I'm grateful for the times I feel comfortable and at ease." When you do this every day, and each time a despairing thought comes up, you will notice a change in your general demeanor. You will feel more hopeful, happy, grateful, and healthful.

6. Finally, take a look back at the notes you made at the beginning of the chapter. How have your thoughts changed after reading this chapter?

Chapter Four

The Life Cycle
of a Doctor

Take Stock of Where You Are Now

Use the following prompts and questions to review your experiences
with your doctors and your treatment history.

1. Advocating for yourself with your medical team is much easier
    when you have documentation. If you've never made a list of
    all of your symptoms, treatments, medications, side effects, tests
    and diagnoses, do so now. Even if you've done it before, consider
    doing it again, here and now, all in one place, as chances are it
    will help you feel empowered and newly focused about what it
    is that you have to manage every day. Simply write the headings
    for each category ("Symptoms," "Treatments," "Medications")
    and scribble away off the top of your head, or, if you feel called

to do so, you may want to create a more systematic and detailed overview using a spreadsheet on your computer.

2. If you haven't done so already, consider requesting all medical records from your present and past medical practitioners. Have a dedicated binder (perhaps buy yourself a beautiful new set) to keep them all together and organized. Prescriptions often come with an extra sticker attached to the information sheet, so you could put a sticker from each medication on a page in your journal or binder and write notes about any side effects or reactions you have as they occur. This practice recently saved a dear friend of mine from taking a medication that had caused her to have a heart attack a year before. Initially she had been confused because it was being referred to by its generic name. Thankfully, when she checked her records, she was able to prove that she should not take that medication and thereby prevented a potential disaster.

3. Using your journal, reflect on your experiences with doctors and other medical professionals. Do you find them to be generally positive or negative? Make a list of all of the positive experiences with healthcare professionals (ones that were perhaps marked by particularly supportive or kind interactions) and all the negative ones (those where you might have experienced doubt and suspicion, for example).

4. If you've ever had to stand up for yourself to a doctor, how did it feel? What did you learn from that experience?

The Wonderful Pieces of Divinity
I Have Found

Trust your instincts; listen to your body,

it will not lie to you.

·

This disease isn't nice; you deserve to be

treated with respect by your doctors.

·

Being your own advocate is empowering.

·

Anger is appropriate sometimes.

·

Know when to say goodbye to a doctor.

Doctors. Sometimes you can't stand them, but you can't live without them. Some are nice and genuinely want to help make you better, while others . . . well, seem to be there to fill up space. A pattern I've noticed, that applies at least to me, is that the life cycle of a specialist for treating a patient with a chronic condition is between two and three years. After that, they seem to run out of patience with me, or I do with them.

Doctors have a hard job. There are so many factors that go into a diagnosis, even for simple things. Chronic and degenerative diseases like autoimmunity are so complicated that it can be almost impossible to diagnose and treat them. Here are a few of the issues I have encountered either simultaneously or at intervals.

Early on, a life-long sensitive stomach turned into an inability to keep anything down. Tests were inconclusive, and I was put on medications to slow digestion and to address the pain.

Next, I had a patch of dry, painful skin on my upper leg. My body—especially my skin—was sensitive and reactive since childhood, and I've heard this echoed by many fellow autoimmune disease patients. When I was little, I used to get dry lips in the winter, and my mouth would swell up like a blowfish. Mom says that when I had chicken pox, I didn't just get chicken pox; I got chicken pox *on top of* my chicken pox.

If I used a new shampoo or facial wash, my whole face would swell, and I would look like a monkey for days. When Mom changed laundry detergents, I would develop hives that would itch, burn, and ooze. I have a rash on my legs, since I was nine years old, that never goes away. It looks like ingrown hairs, except without the ingrown hair part; no one ever seemed to know why.

After I assured the doctor several times that I wasn't sexually active and it couldn't be an STD, he decided it was some sort of heat rash or eczema and prescribed a cream. The cream didn't help.

When I got mononucleosis (mono) the doctor gave me Cefzil, an antibiotic, thinking it was strep throat (not a bad guess because I had strep multiple times per year). Within a day or so, I began to swell up all over my body and then, on top of the swelling, red blotches and dots began forming. My throat was constricted, and my voice sounded like I was talking through a tube. My eyes swelled shut. I scratched in my sleep until I bled. I took oatmeal baths, put on calamine lotion, and took antihistamines. I couldn't get any relief. Eventually, they realized the infection was mono instead of strep and the antibiotic and mono were reacting to each other, causing the rash. They promptly took me off of the antibiotic, but it still took tons of steroids, antihistamines, and a couple of weeks for the reaction to subside.

It appears the mono, and possibly the immune system/allergic reason between the drug and the mono, were the catalysts for my immune system to trip the switch from normal to self-attacking. Thus began, smack in the middle of my college years, the long parade of doctors coming in and out of my life.

Seeing Lots of Doctors Is Part of It

How many doctors do "normal" people see? If you see a doctor on a yearly basis, with sporadic visits in between, you might change general practitioners every few years as insurance changes, you move, or your doctor's availability becomes less convenient. You may have regular appointments for preventative dental and eye care. You may even have a specialist here and there, as certain situations arise. The choice of a doctor works a little differently for someone with a chronic condition.

We each have an extensive list of specialists. I currently have a rheumatologist, neurologist, dermatologist, retina specialist, gastroenterologist, and physical therapist. Those are in addition to my general practitioner, gynecologist, dentist, and optometrist.

It can be a full time challenge balancing all of these specialists. As I write this, I notice I haven't seen my gastroenterologist in over a year, I'm six months overdue on my well-woman check-up, and I am two months late on my dental cleaning.

My schedule is filled with appointments but not for fun things like meetups and lunches with friends. We're talking about tests, blood work, and doctor's appointments that are two hours long (or rather, that consist of 105 minutes of waiting and fifteen minutes with the doc, but who's counting?).

Expect Frustration and Resentment

What happens when you have been seeing a doctor for a while, say two or three years, and he or she gets tired of hearing the same thing from you over and over? What happens when, despite their best efforts, doctors are unable to help you get better? Frustration and resentment abound.

Doctors are human, and if they are not seeing any progress in your health, they may become frustrated as well. This is understandable. Still, I have often wanted to shake my doctors and say, "Who are you to be testy with me? It's my life that is at risk!"

At a certain point I feel like some doctors try the same thing (drug, treatment, etc.) over and over, expecting a different result. This is not only futile but the famous definition of insanity.

What's worse is when you can tell that the doctor has stopped listening to you about your symptoms and is only hearing what he or she wants or expects to hear; or, worse yet, he or she is dismissing your concerns outright.

I have lived with a symptom (severely weakened hand/arm strength and stamina) for over a year, telling a specific doctor about it on each quarterly appointment. These symptoms affect my daily functioning. Small and major motor skills are equally affected. Opening doorknobs, carrying groceries, and lifting heavy objects all become impossible tasks.

A typical question in my day-to-day life is: How many hours does it take to change a light bulb? That depends; is a neighbor home? No, well I'm not climbing a ladder alone, and I can't grip the little bolt to unscrew the fixture. Even if I did, I'll probably find a way to burn myself on the hot bulb or drop it with my slippery fingers and/or cut myself on broken glass. So it's better to sit in the dark for the next eight hours until Scott gets home and let him change it. It's a good time to meditate.

This particular doctor dismissed the symptom, saying it didn't appear to be a problem to her, even after testing my strength through the squeeze test. As I explained how the weakened hands manifested in real life (that it wasn't initial strength but two to three seconds into the exertion), she stood by her assessment rather than listening to how it hindered my life.

When I saw my old Mayo Clinic doctor again, I was assured this hand/arm condition was, in fact, not normal or something to ignore, nor was it something that I should have to live with. He ran blood work and an EMG to determine if it was a new development or just deconditioning. Once the tests were determined to be normal—and I was actually in remission—he decided that through physical therapy and swimming I might regain some of the lost strength and stamina in my hands and wrists.

These little things—listening to the patient instead of just making assumptions—make all the difference in our lives. I may never get all of my hand strength back, or maybe I will. But having the opportunity to try is a heck of a lot better than having my concerns dismissed.

Do You Have Drug Allergies?

Another thing people with autoimmunity might have in common is drug allergies. I am allergic to a lot of them, and when doctors and nurses see my list, they often comment on the length. I also have sensitivities, as opposed to outright allergies, to some drugs, meaning that while I can take them, I have to be careful because my reaction can go from a mild sensitivity to a full blown allergic reaction at any point.

Prednisone, a steroid, is often the first line drug of choice for autoimmunity. I have been on many different doses of it over the years. However, there is a fine line, or threshold, of how many milligrams I can take. Over the last five years or so, my threshold has been five milligrams per day. That means that until recently, I hadn't been successful in getting below five milligrams; I am also not able to go above that level for even two days. If I do take more than this amount, I have hot, crushing, grinding leg and hip pain that takes my breath away and renders me unable to walk normally. I had an x-ray to check for necrosis, and it was negative. Therefore, the pain remains unexplained, except for the direct correlation between increasing the prednisone and the onset of pain.

I tell every new doctor I see that this happens, and I make it clear that I will not go above five milligrams of prednisone. They nod and act like they have heard all of this before. But the first time they see me have a flare-up, they invariably talk about increasing prednisone.

Since I can't expect them to remember my issues with the white-hot, grinding pain, I kindly remind them that I do not take more than five milligrams and why. Then I watch as gentle, sympathetic helpfulness turns to anger, indignation, and then passive acceptance. They suspect I am one of those medically noncompliant patients who will argue with them about my treatment.

Your Doctor Is Not Always Right

It can be amusing to watch these emotions play out on their faces and, given my extensive experience with prior doctors, I can usually guess what they are thinking. In the past I have allowed them to intimidate me into upping the dosage. Without fail, I end up calling them back two or three days later. Through clenched teeth, I tell them the pain is happening again and beg for help to undo the damage the prednisone increase has done.

Not anymore. I've stopped caring whether doctors label me as noncompliant, or even as a bitch. I'm not taking more than five milligrams period; the pain isn't worth it. Doctors don't always know best. I maintain respect and cordiality, but I stand up for myself when I need to. After all, I know my body best.

Depression can be a four-letter word to a person with auto-immunity. One of the most detrimental misdiagnoses doctors made repeatedly over the years when they were stumped by my condition was to dismiss me as psychosomatic, or label my physical symptoms as signs of depression.

These labels got my treatment nowhere and caused me much emotional pain. It made me question everything I knew about myself. I was quiet and had rough patches, yes, but with my decision to be more outgoing, I had really turned myself into a happy, look-at-the-bright-side-of-life kind of gal. I had many friends, enjoyed life, and always had a smile on my face.

Even so, there I was at twenty-two years old—unable to walk normally, having physical trouble getting out of bed because of pain, and taking Darvocet every four hours without complete relief. I begged for help, and the doctors continued to treat me with anti-depressants while acting like nothing was physically wrong. Never mind the positive antinuclear antibodies (ANAs) and other blood work. There were even a couple of doctors who thought they could attribute all of my symptoms to drug-seeking behavior, depression, and lack of sleep.

Mind you, I have never exhibited drug-seeking behavior. The extent of my mind-altering activity was the occasional alcohol consumption. I hated how the Darvocet made me feel, but if I didn't take it, the pain was so much worse. While there is a history of depression in my family, my symptoms were so clearly physical that I was incredulous a doctor would minimize my experience in such a manner.

I have experienced bouts of depression. When you have a chronic disease and your body is out of control, depression seems to come along and say "hello" periodically. I found that when doctors get lost in my diagnosis, when they stop having answers and feel helpless to know how to treat me, they begin throwing around the "D-word."

It's Okay and Normal to Experience Depression

I wouldn't have a problem with the word "depression" if it were addressed as an episodic condition brought on by the flare-ups of the disease, and not as a chronic condition. Unfortunately, when a doctor says, "I think you are depressed," it brings back the years of feeling minimized, unheard, and untreated by the doctors. It takes me back to the time when they wanted to dismiss my symptoms as being all in my head and manifestations of some sort of mental illness, rather than a physical condition.

I have a support system that I trust to tell me the truth. I can ask its members, "Am I just being gloomy, or is this sadness getting to the point that I need help?" Sometimes the answer was that I needed to find help getting out of my hole of sadness, and other times it was just a matter of time or perspective.

In January 2013, I had a crazy round of illnesses. In the space of six weeks I had a minor respiratory infection, my fourteenth case of shingles, my fourth retinal detachment, another bout of shingles brought on by the stress of surgery, and influenza A. Finally, after getting over the ten days of Tamiflu, I got another cold.

Coincidentally, I had an appointment with one of my disease specialists right around that time. After hearing about all of my sicknesses in the previous weeks and my fears that I might be headed for a worsening of my disease, she asked, "How are you sleeping?" My answer was, "I am not sleeping well." She didn't ask if my sleep disturbance was new. If she had, the answer would've been, "No, I've had insomnia for twenty years."

Instead, she proceeded with what her agenda was from the start of the conversation when she saw I was crying. She didn't reply with empathy, comfort, or a plan about how she would help me get through it if a flare-up occurred.

Does Any of This Sound Familiar?

You may have experienced a moment with a doctor like the one I was about to have. It's like being sucked out of your body and into the twilight zone. Things go hazy and surreal. You get lightheaded; you feel like maybe you are losing your grip on reality even though you know you are not. Have you been there? The following is what happened in that moment.

I was crying out of desperation as I talked about the six things that had recently gone wrong with my body. Who wouldn't be crying?

Instead of responding with a proactive plan to keep me from having another flare-up, she looked me in the eye and said, "You're depressed. You need an antidepressant."

Screech—wait—what?

Did she just dismiss nearly two months of illnesses—including surgery—as insignificant and, instead, diagnose me with depression, without asking me any questions about my life, about my marriage, or about my coping mechanisms?

"I'm sorry, I must have misunderstood. Did you understand when I gave a detailed description of all the infections, the surgery, etc.?"

"Yes, I did, and I don't think you are flaring; I think you are depressed. Are you against taking antidepressants?" she asked accusingly.

I replied, "Well, no, of course not. I have taken them before. I just don't understand what depression has to do with my body, and the recurring *physical stressors*."

"I don't think you are *handling* things well, and not sleeping is an indication of depression. I think you should take antidepressants, and you will feel better."

My thoughts went wild. I got confused and a little angry because I thought this doctor was a specialist in my disease. I didn't know she thought she was a psychiatrist. I have taken antidepressants before when my disease flared, and being sick and out of control of my health made me depressed, but it was only for a short period of time. I thought I'd give her the benefit of the doubt; maybe she was only talking about a couple of months. In that case, maybe it wouldn't hurt. I tried not to feel pushed back to the pre-diagnosis years when doctors accused me of being a hypochondriac because they couldn't come up with a diagnosis. I hadn't slept well in over twenty years and hadn't been depressed that long. *Take a deep breath*, I told myself, *in and out. Okay, are you ready? Yes? Okay. Let's try this again. Ever the kind patient.*

"If I agree to take it, how long are you thinking I should be on it?"

"A year."

I wanted to say, "No way! I have a beautiful life! I have a wonderful, supportive husband and a perfectly healthy child. *If* I am depressed, it is because my body feels like dung warmed over. I have a two- maybe three-month-long depression brought on by my body, my disease, multiple infections, and surgery—not a yearlong depression. Here's an idea, lady: Why don't you fix my body, and then I won't have any need to feel depressed whatsoever! How's that?"

Instead I said, "Okay, thank you," and left as quickly as I could.

Don't Be Afraid to Change Doctors

Back in the car, I called my husband sobbing and asked if he thought I was depressed. He said, "No, I think you're sick, why?" I told him the story, and he said, "That's ridiculous, she doesn't know you. I guess it's time for a new rheumatologist." I called one of my best friends and asked her the same questions, and she followed with the same answers. I didn't fill the prescription.

I called around the next day to find a new doctor, having lost my trust in her ability to treat my disease, and that's how I found out my old Mayo Clinic doctor was now only a four hour drive away.

This is just one narrative of many like it. I have heard many stories of patients with chronic diseases being treated similarly, and I've witnessed others go through analogous experiences. Once when I was in the hospital, I shared a room with a woman with an autoimmune disease. I believe it was scleroderma. I listened to how the doctors talked to her, how dismissive they were of her pain, and how patronizing they were.

She was in a lot of pain. She complained a lot, and it was probably annoying them. But you know what? It was their job to listen to her and to help her, no matter their personal opinions of her. She didn't choose to be in pain. I am sure she just wanted compassion, relief from her pain, and perhaps a little bit of hope. I would guess she left that hospital feeling a little more demoralized, less valued, and definitely not heard by the doctors.

We deserve—as patients and human beings—more than dismissive behavior from the doctors charged with our care.

I don't wish this disease on anyone. I do, however, wish doctors would learn to be more empathetic. Have you heard of those labor simulators that partners of pregnant women can wear to get an idea of what childbirth feels like? It's too bad they don't have something like that for doctors dealing with patients with chronic diseases. Can you imagine your doctor walking around in an "Autoimmunity Simulator 5000?"

The Challenge of Looking "Well"

One of the challenges of having autoimmunity is that, most of the time, we look pretty normal. We may have rashes and redness, and we may walk a little differently, slower and more labored, but for the most part, we blend in with the healthy crowd.

If I could teach doctors anything it would be that our pain, muscle weakness, shortness of breath, skin sensitivity, and voluminous lists of other symptoms are no less painful, or less real, just because they cannot see them. We ache for a normal life. We yearn to run and play with our kids like others do. We wish we could stop hurting. We would love for our string of doctor visits to be a distant memory.

We live in our bodies twenty-four hours a day, 365 days a year. You may know how to translate symptoms into medical jargon, but don't forget that we are the actual experts on our own bodies. We know when something is not right and when something has changed. Our very ability to get around in the world depends on being able to listen to, read, and accommodate the signals our bodies send us. To survive, we have become attuned to things in our bodies that others could not imagine. Listen to us; we *know* what we're talking about.

If doctors and patients are both working toward the same goal—the patient's health—where does it go wrong?

Now, to Be Fair . . .

Do doctors wake up one day and say, "I have seen this patient for 'X' number of months or years, so I will stop listening to him or her"? No, of course not. But, like everyone else, they have egos, and they get frustrated when they aren't making a difference with our symptoms. They might forget that no matter how frustrating it is to treat autoimmune diseases, it is nothing compared to the exasperation and heartbreak involved in actually living with one.

It *is* possible that in their mind, patients start to run together and become dehumanized, as doctors are pushed to meet with a certain number of patients per day, fill out requisite paperwork, and do whatever else they have to do. They may get tired of hearing one patient after another whine and complain.

Be Fair to Yourself, Too

When I start to get that feeling—you know, the one you get when you are dating someone and he or she is more interested in the wallpaper than in the conversation you are having—or, in this case, the feeling that my doctor is just not that into me anymore? That's when I know it's time to move on and find a new doctor.

I learned a long time ago that I can't put my life and the health of my body into the hands of a disinterested doctor. I hope you share the same sense of inner strength.

Creative Tips for Empowering Yourself

- Bring a list of questions and concerns to your doctor's visit so that you don't get flustered, forgetting what you wanted to say; also take a pen and paper to the appointment so you can make notes.

- Ask a trusted friend or family member to accompany you. They can be an advocate for you and also help you remember the conversation and instructions.

- If a doctor is rude, remember they are human, and it's not personal. However, that doesn't mean you have to continue using him or her as your practitioner.

- Repeat after me: "I deserve respect. I have the right to be heard, to assert myself, to participate in my medical decisions, and to have my questions answered. If I feel these needs aren't being met, I have the right to seek out a new practitioner."

Caregiver Tips

- Consider accompanying your loved one to appointments if he or she is willing. The emotional support is invaluable, and when a doctor is being difficult, it helps to have back up.

- Never minimize your loved one's experience, even when the doctors do. You may look at your loved one and think he or she doesn't look sick, but please don't say that. Until you have walked in your loved one's shoes, you cannot imagine the amount of pain, weakness, and fatigue he or she experiences. By showing support and compassion, you acknowledge the experience, even if you do not understand it, allowing your loved one to feel safe despite what the doctors say.

Create Your Own Marvelous Transformation

Time for reflection and integration. Let the following questions and prompts guide you as you write down your responses in your journal.

1. What situation or example resonated most with you in this chapter?

2. When faced with similar situations, how do you feel, act, or think?

3. What would you most like to remember from this chapter?

4. If you should encounter an uncooperative doctor in the future, what will you do differently now than you would have done before?

5. State in one or two declarative sentences how you feel, now, about your right to being respected.

6. Make a list of the top ten most important behaviors and attitudes you want to see from a doctor. Once you've completed the list, consider to what extent your current medical team is meeting these expectations. If any of them fall short, are you open to considering getting a second opinion, or even finding a new doctor?

7. Look back at the notes you made before you read the chapter. How have your thoughts changed after reading this chapter?

Chapter Five

The Ups
and Downs

Take Stock of Where You Are Now

Take some time to look at your experiences of the emotional roller coaster that is living with a chronic disease. Write in your journal, and let the following questions guide you.

1. What are the most significant ups and downs you experienced with your disease?

2. If you've had a time when you thought your symptoms were under control only to be surprised by a flare-up, write a short paragraph about it. How did that make you feel physically? Emotionally? Spiritually?

3. Think back and try to remember a time during which you felt like nothing would go right and then a time when you ever

felt like you were on top of it all and ready to take on the world.

4. If you've ever taken extreme measures to try to get well ("extreme" being a relative term), such as taken a chance on experimental or alternative treatments, describe how it felt to take that little bit of control over your situation. If you've never done something like that, describe the fears that are holding you back.

5. If you ever feel alone, and like no one understands what you are going through, what do you currently do to help yourself feel better?

The Wonderful Pieces of Divinity I Have Found

There *are* doctors and nurses who really do care, who will be your advocates, and help you get better.

·

Be thankful for the medications that *do* work.

·

There is no such thing as "fair"; take a deep breath.

·

Counting your blessings will help you overcome that sense of unfairness.

·

Successes, even if short-lived or intermittent, are still successes; strive to accomplish them.

·

You didn't do anything to deserve this; there is no one to blame. Stop feeling guilty about being sick.

In 2008 I had five surgeries. A close friend had sworn to me that this was going to be my year. That after all the time of being sick, she was sure I was about to turn it all around. And I'd bought it. *Mind over matter*, I thought, *I am ready for a change!* It didn't quite play out that way. Many people with autoimmunity experience these letdowns—a time when they thought their health was improving, only to be disappointed by a new mountain (and not a mere bump) in the road.

The craziness of that year started on January 2, when I went for a routine eye exam. With absolutely no warning or prior signs, the ophthalmologist found I had a full retinal detachment in one eye and lattice detachment in the other. I had double eye surgery the very next day, needing the placement of a scleral buckle on one eye and laser surgery on the other.

Three weeks after the eye surgeries I had a tonsillectomy, followed by a miscarriage and a D&C (Dilation and Curettage, a cervical procedure) in July, followed by another eye surgery, and, finally, a hysterectomy in October.

The year took an emotional toll. It went from being "my year" to "my year of surgeries," as we now jokingly call it. It was stressful and demoralizing—especially considering that the second miscarriage (I'd had my first one the year before) led to the decision to give up the possibility of having another baby. Prior to 2008, the only surgery I'd had was my C-section, a required procedure given the state of my health, but one with a priceless outcome. I'd considered myself lucky to have made it to thirty-one with only one surgery. Now I made up for it all in the course of one year, beginning to feel like Cavity Sam from the game Operation. Every time I "went under" I felt more out of control of my body.

All of that physical and emotional stress affected my body and the disease in such a way that when 2009 dawned, I noticed I could no longer lift my daughter—just three-years old at the time and a tiny sprite—without straining. I had progressively more trouble holding my arms above my head to brush my hair, my hips were going out more and more often, and my skin became more red and inflamed than it had ever been.

Don't Hesitate to Make a Major Move

By the end of 2009 we were through playing around. Scott and I both felt we weren't getting anywhere with the doctors I was seeing, and a friend recommended we look into visiting the Mayo Clinic. We were told the physicians there might know of cutting-edge treatments local doctors hadn't considered. Within weeks we scheduled my first appointment in Scottsdale, Arizona.

That's another characteristic common to people suffering from a chronic disease like autoimmunity: We are willing to go to the ends of the earth to get the help we need. I live in St. Louis, Missouri, and traveled to Scottsdale, Arizona, three times in one year to visit the Mayo Clinic.

The Mayo Clinic provided the most positive healthcare experience I'd ever had. For once I really felt heard (the beautiful weather, scenery, and visits with family and friends certainly contributed). The rheumatologist took over my care and coordinated testing that would not only verify my diagnosis but also assess the progression and status of the disease.

These things had not been priorities to my doctors at home, yet now they were being done and seemed obvious and important. I expressed my frustration with the medications I received at home, my lack of progress, and my fear that if I was this bad at age thirty-three, I didn't have much further to deteriorate.

The attending physician assured me he was there to help, and we would make a plan. The following January, I returned for results (and a biopsy), and he recommended a course of intravenous immunoglobulin (IVIG) treatments to stall and possibly even reverse my disease, followed by methotrexate to manage it going forward.

Stall and reverse? I hadn't known this was even a possibility! It was only ever about how to maintain or prevent further decline. For the first time in years, I had hope.

Are You Open to New or Novel Treatments?

IVIG is an infusion of the immune cells from the blood of thousands of donors mixed into one bottle that is fed into the body. From what I understand, it has the potential to be effective against a great many diseases, and autoimmunity is high on the list. It appears to work by replacing or overriding a person's own immune system, thereby keeping it from attacking the body. However, getting insurance companies to approve IVIG treatments is difficult because of the costs involved.

I went home in January and started my twelve-month course of IVIG. As the medicine flowed into my veins, I pictured it repairing my body, replacing damaged cells, and coating my frayed nerves.

You may have seen the dynamic visual effects in the television show *House,* when a camera takes you through a vein into an organ to show how a medication enters the blood stream and works its wonders. I envisioned IVIG flowing through my veins like that, encasing and flushing out bad cells, sealing muscle tears, rebuilding fibers, and turning reddened skin back to white. I encouraged my body to soak it in and take full advantage of its healing powers.

It worked; I felt 50 percent better within a week.

Instead of spiraling toward certain disability, I began climbing out of the dark hole of sickness. Along the way I encountered some of the sweetest, most caring, and compassionate nurses I have ever met. On the whole, during those twelve months I was the healthiest, strongest, most vibrant person I had ever experienced myself being.

We called my monthly infusions my "liquid gold," because of the enormous cost—in excess of $20,000 a month—and because I could feel my body healing, as this precious liquid gold pumped through my veins.

One day, about three months into treatment, my daughter dropped a toy between the cushions of our sofa. There I was lying on the floor—the woman who had barely been able to lift her thirty-pound daughter three months earlier—when super-human strength came over me. From that prone position, I lifted the sofa with one hand, reached in, and grabbed the toy. I had put it back down before I realized what I had done. In that moment I felt like I could climb Mount Everest, when just weeks before I could barely climb the stairs.

I am known for being a klutz, partly because I tend to have my head in the clouds but also due to a condition called "foot drop." In other words, I fall a lot. I've had three crowns put on my front tooth because, on the way down, I seem to lead with my mouth.

One of the more memorable clumsiness incidents occurred the last night in the Puget Sound during our honeymoon. We were walking back to our bed-and-breakfast after dinner when I misjudged a curb and face planted. Glasses got bent, eyes were blackened, and my nose and front crown were broken.

One ambulance ride and an emergency room visit later, the nice paramedics had been able to put humpty dumpty back together again, albeit with some tape and gauze. We made our early morning flight where my jack-o'-lantern smile was a hit on the plane, as Scott and I laughed our way through the whole thing. My face, including a new crown, was back in order before long, but it's memories like these that highlight what an accomplishment my next milestone truly was.

Thanks to the IVIG, I was able to start running for the first time since childhood. Weak hips and trunk muscles had always made it impossible to run or jump, but as I became stronger I wanted to give it a try. The first few times I ran, I managed only four steps before getting exhausted and having to walk. But eventually I worked up to running six-mile stretches without any breaks. *Hooray*!

What I really did was jog—other people could walk and keep up with me—but it didn't matter. I was moving in a way that jostled my body, and it felt great.

I took full advantage of the year of my IVIG treatments and ran a few times a week. But once the treatment was over and the liquid gold left my body, the super-human strength disappeared. I have maintained some of my overall health, but I am no longer able to run. I miss it.

Those months of running were a gift: feeling the pavement beneath my pounding feet, feeling the wind whip around my face, the sweat drip down my back. Some day I might be able to do that again, but if not, I am still thankful I had that wonderful experience for a brief time.

Be Sure to Monitor Your Side Effects

IVIG is not without its drawbacks—in my case the side effects. Every infusion contained Benadryl, Tylenol, and Zofran as well as migraine medicine as preventatives. I would still get spinal headaches of a magnitude that made my prior migraines seem like mosquito bites. During the infusions I would feel like I was being tossed in a dinghy on a violent ocean—motion sickness. The surges would be so forceful I'd almost fall out of my chair.

There is always the risk of a dangerous allergic reaction to IVIG called aseptic meningitis (AM). My side effects could have indicated AM, but I refused to go to the ER to be checked for it. I was so desperate to have my liquid gold that, under my doctor's guidance, we allowed for this possibility. We slowed my dosing, monitored my vitals, and I would sleep through the infusion to avoid feeling a lot of it.

For days I would walk around with headaches, muscle aches, constipation, dizziness, slowed reaction time, and various other symptoms. I got resourceful and found ways to deal with the side effects. I discovered that froufrou coffee drinks with a lot of cream helped with the tummy issues. Greasy burgers helped with the nausea, and ice packs on my neck helped slightly with the headaches.

In 2012 I received another four-month round of liquid gold, then transitioned from one immunosuppressant drug— methotrexate, which caused a side effect of thrush so bad my throat almost closed—to another, CellCept. The surge of strength wasn't quite as big this time; it was a different brand and also didn't have the same intensity of side effects.

The transition between medications went well, and I have maintained decent health on CellCept for over a year now without any major flares. In fact, it's been going so well that I'm currently being weaned off CellCept and prednisone. Despite multiple infections in the first half of this year, the disease has remained in check.

You're Not Alone

With all the loving support in the world, my situation still feels cruelly unfair sometimes. It's all well and good to try to find the best in each situation, but the truth is that sometimes I want to scream and shout, "This is not fair! I didn't do anything to deserve this! I'm a nice person! I take care of myself. I'm a loving mom and wife. Why has my body, my life, my God, and my self, forsaken me? Why me?"

These are feelings of frustration, indignation, and resentment, and they deserve to be acknowledged. The occasional outbursts are okay, perhaps even good for me, because those moments allow me to get it out and start fresh. If you've ever been overcome by these feelings, I hope this book will at least let you know that you are not alone.

There is no such thing as "fair." We are all here on our own journey, and life is simply what we make of our experience. When I get bogged down in the unfairness of it all, I count my blessings. I am still here and relatively healthy; I could have things that are much worse; I have a roof over my head, a supportive husband, a sweet daughter, and the list goes on and on. I have come to understand that fair is another four-letter word. It makes me feel defeated and cheated. I have tried to replace it with action.

Just when I thought I couldn't get any better, I ran six miles. Just when I think I can't push on any more, I look at my family and realize that I *cannot* stop fighting. Just when I feel all hope is lost, someone has a new idea, treatment, or modality to try.

"Letting Go" Is a Marvelous Tool

I didn't do anything to deserve this; *neither did you!* No one does. Autoimmunity is a combination of genetics and environment. There is no cosmic retribution or karma that brought it on. It is purely a matter of biology meeting environmental stimuli.

My world changed when I accepted this fact. I let go of the guilt and pain that had come out of the feeling that I wasn't a good enough person to be healthy. I let go of notions that somehow my body, God, or my self were betraying me. In doing so, I found that I felt better, happier, lighter, and more in control of my life.

Maybe by taking that leap of acceptance you can see your world change, too.

Creative Tips for Empowering Yourself

- Set goals with reasonable milestones, and celebrate little achievements along the way. Would walking to the mailbox unassisted be a huge accomplishment for you? Then start by walking five steps a day. Do you want to swim laps? Start by treading water and dog paddling. Do you want to cook a meal? Start by standing long enough to fry an egg. As you build up strength, make the activity longer.

· Medications are there to help us, and they serve a wonderful purpose. When you take your meds, picture them doing their work and thank them for the relief they are about to provide.

· Remove the word "fair" from your vocabulary; it diminishes your power by allowing you to feel like a victim. If you replace it with "willful action," you can see your world change before your eyes.

· Repeat after me: "I am not a victim. My condition is not a reflection of who I am. I am whole just the way I am."

Caregiver Tips

· Be willing to advocate for your loved one within your means. If that means getting a second opinion when things are not going well, you can show your support by assisting in arranging that.

· When things keep going wrong, don't judge your loved one, cast blame, or doubt his or her sincerity; he or she feels overwhelmed and stupid enough when one thing after another goes wrong. What your loved one needs from you is unconditional support and love, not doubt or judgment.

Create Your Own Marvelous Transformation

Take some time to reflect on what you've read and to solidify any positive realizations you may have had. In your journal, respond to the following questions.

1. What situation or example resonated most with you in this chapter?

2. When faced with similar situations, how do you feel, act, or think?

3. What would you most like to remember from this chapter?

4. How do you now feel about thinking outside the box when it comes to treatments? What, if anything, has changed?

5. How do you now feel about being alone with your disease? What comfort can you derive from knowing there are others like you?

6. Describe what it means for you to challenge yourself—emotionally, physically, and spiritually?

7. What major emotion did you sense coming from me, the author, in this chapter? What emotion did that spark for you? What can you learn from your reaction to my story?

8. What do you think you can now do to feel less alone? Who, in your community, can you rely on for emotional support? Make a list of those people, and make sure you have all of their contact information readily available. Consider finding new ways to connect with these significant contacts and to strengthen your bond. For example, if you tend to speak over the phone,

consider meeting up in person. If you've only ever connected via social media, consider speaking via Skype, or writing a good old-fashioned letter. If you have friends or acquaintances you haven't connected with online, consider reaching out to them in that format. An existing relationship can be enriched by an online connection, too.

9. Finally, look back at the notes you made before you read the chapter. How have your thoughts changed?

Chapter Six

I Am a
Cartoon Character

Take Stock of Where You Are Now

Consider the following three questions and respond to each briefly in your journal.

1. When everything seems to go wrong, how do you cope? Do you find humor in your situation? Or do you get down, feel that effort is futile, and want to give up? Think of and describe the three funniest things that have happened in your illness experience. Now think of and write down the three most upsetting things that have happened to you due to your illness.

2. Do you ever feel as though you are making it all up? That things can't possibly get *this bad*? Do you encounter skepticism from

your family and friends? Write a few sentences about how these questions make you feel.

3. Do you ever just want to scream and cry about the unfairness of it all? Do you ever think, "Why me?"

4. In a few words, respond to the question, Do you feel guilty or ashamed for being sick?

The Wonderful Pieces of Divinity I Have Found

Humor can save your life.

·

Don't hold it all in, all of the time.

·

Allow yourself to be vulnerable.

·

Be thankful for your support system;
they keep you going when you want to quit.

·

Take good care of yourself.

·

Incidents that seem negative
can have positive outcomes.

Sometimes I feel like a cartoon character—Wile E. Coyote, to be exact—standing on the edge of a cliff:

- I freeze in motion, and there's a piano about to drop on my head—that is dermatomyositis;

- an anvil is about to hit my face—retinal detachment;

- an arrow is aimed at my chest—recurrent shingles;

- a truck is bearing down on me—chronic migraines;

- a clock is clanging next to my ear—insomnia;

- a metal vice vibrates around my waist—fibromyalgia;

- hot coals are pelted at my stomach—Irritable Bowel Syndrome (IBS);

- the crack in the ledge I'm standing on—influenza; and so on.

Autoimmunity is hard to diagnose because so many conditions and diseases mimic each other. Autoimmunity is also still a misunderstood and complex process; the medical profession hasn't yet figured out how everything works together. This is the reason why patients end up with so many layers of diagnoses.

I am, basically, a mess—as can be deduced from the list of ailments and diagnoses I've already shared ad nauseam. I never understood how science has sent a man to the moon but can't figure out how to connect the majority of these symptoms. It seems intuitive to me that many of them are interrelated but, so far, many of the connections have not been made.

Is Anyone Looking for Links?

For example, it hasn't been proven that people with dermatomyositis are at higher risk for recurrent retinal detachments. Retinas are made of skin and connective tissue, and dermatomyositis attacks skin and muscles. I have also developed macular scar tissue, or a macular pucker, which is a fairly rare condition. However, doctor after doctor has told me there is no connection between them.

Also, you'd think someone could find a link between the chronic migraines and dermatomyositis, especially since lupus and migraines appear to be linked.

Migraines started occurring simultaneously with the onset of my disease, but there is no evidence of a link. If they aren't related, it makes it seem even more unfair. Migraines are debilitating. I've been told over and over again that they are completely unrelated to dermatomyositis, but my experience informs me otherwise: migraines stem from the alternating weakness and muscle tightening in my neck. They are less prevalent when my dermatomyositis is less active and more prevalent when I have a flare up. I see auras and have light sensitivity. There is pain that I would describe as grinding, stabbing, and/or crushing. The slightest movement in my pinky can feel like a 9.5 magnitude earthquake. It always results in a migraine-like hangover the next day.

Blood vessels in my face and forehead often burst, and my scalp and face can get tingly, tender, and raw during and following an episode. They are also accompanied by nausea.

Using the process of elimination, I have narrowed down the causes over the years. Eating the wrong things or physical strain, particularly in the neck area, can cause them. Changes in the weather, such as barometric pressures dropping or rising rapidly, rainstorms, snowstorms, changes in humidity, and extreme fluctuation in temperature—pretty much any unsettledness in the atmosphere can bring them about.

Are There Possible Remedies for Your Migraines?

A bad migraine can put me in bed for two to three days unable to move. For a while I was getting hit by one of those every week. I've tried a number of methods to prevent them, including heart medication, Botox injections, massages, antihistamines, and muscles relaxers, not to mention all of the rescue meds. While some of them worked for short periods of time, none of them lasted long.

At the end of 2012, the doctor recommended I try Topamax. I went from multiple bedridden days a week to just one headache a week, and sometimes none at all. The new "bad" means that light hurts, but I can go about my day—slower than normal, but I can get out of bed. Gradually, through natural remedies (vitamins, herbal formulas, and essential oils), I decreased them even more and was able to begin decreasing the Topamax; hopefully that cycle is broken.

Once I solved one issue (migraines), another would appear. It wasn't two weeks after seeing some relief from the Topamax before I was hit with weeks of infections, shingles, and retinal detachment. It was the day before my eye surgery, after dropping off our daughter at my mom's house, when I turned to my husband in the car and gave him the cartoon character analogy for the first time.

Expect Occasional Meltdowns

After saying goodbye to my daughter, and on my way to another surgery, I lost it. Overwhelmed, I told Scott I wasn't sure how much more of this I could take or how much more of it I really *wanted* to take. I told him the only thing that keeps me holding on is being a wife and a mom; I was tired of the ups and downs and tired of getting one thing fixed only to have three more pop up. The possibility that this time my retina would detach to the point that my doctor wouldn't be able to save my eye frightened me to death. I was so tired of it all, and just sick of being sick.

I felt like no one, not even my beloved Scott, truly understood how hard it was, and how every time something else went wrong I'd feel more beaten down. In that short car ride home, I released all of my pent-up anger, fear, and pain. I couldn't hide it anymore in that moment, the way I usually did in order to protect those around me. Frustrated, I told him that I knew of people who would have committed suicide by now if they were in my position, because the frustration, pain, and futility is just so overwhelming that it feels like there is no way out. No matter what I did, no matter how hard I tried to exercise and eat healthy, my body betrayed me at every turn.

As I sobbed and rocked in my seat, I am sure he didn't know what to do. He listened and let me get it out; when I stopped, he asked what he could do and what I needed from him.

"I don't know," I said.

"I don't know. Maybe don't think I've totally lost it when I lose hope like this. I am just sharing my feelings with you. Maybe just hold me and let me get it out; just allow me to stop being strong for five minutes."

And he did.

How to Find Strength

Waves of anguish can come over you. There are times when you feel hopeless and helpless. But these are also the times when you can come out feeling stronger. With my meltdown, instead of holding it in and allowing it to fester, I purged it; I got it out. Scott being there the way he was—not feeling the need to answer my every sentence but allowing me to be in the space the way I needed to be—was more helpful than if he had tried to problem solve and offer a solution to every statement I made.

Managing a chronic disease is about being strong, but it is also about having the strength to be honest about your limitations and voicing your truth when things get too tough to handle quietly. If you don't have a safe person like Scott who you can vent to, someone who will listen without needing to solve everything, consider turning to your pet, your God, Nature, or a support group.

There are counselors who specialize in chronic conditions. One of the best ways I've found to not let autoimmunity dictate who I am is turning to the wonderful support system around me. I must allow them to help me. I hope you will do the same for yourself.

Bats in My Belfry

In 2013, I had an electromyogram (EMG) to check the muscles and nerves in my arms to determine the cause of their weakness. There was no new damage. That, coupled with recent blood work, led the doctor to say that I had no active muscle disease at the time. In other words, the muscle part of my disease was in remission. The goal then became to wean me off of immunosuppressants. *Yippee!* Two weeks later, what did we find flying around our hundred-year-old house? A flipping bat!

The problem was he could have bitten any one of us, and we wouldn't have known it because the bite marks of bats are like tiny pin pricks. Big deal—ever heard of rabies? When my sister and her batman, I mean friend, came over to get it out of our house, we didn't know we were supposed to keep the bat so it could be tested. I just wanted it out of our house; and so our hero just released the bat outside.

Given the chance of one of us unknowingly having gotten bitten overnight, and due to the fact that we failed to have the bat tested for rabies, it suddenly *was* a big deal. Considering rabies is undetectable in humans until symptoms start, and that once they do start the disease is close to being 100 percent fatal, we arrived at the inevitable conclusion: We all had to get vaccinated for rabies.

I had *just* found out I was in remission after years of fighting my disease. I was looking forward to tapering off meds, and now I had to get some serious rabies vaccinations on the off chance that a bat had bit me (small chance, but possible) and that it had rabies (an even smaller chance but still possible). *Are you kidding me?* Furthermore, I am immunosuppressed dealing with an immune system that doesn't handle anything correctly. Add a big fat syringe to the cartoon and label it "bat."

It gets better. One of the CDC's recommendations involves the issue of whether or not you can take immunosuppressants while receiving the rabies vaccines. They say you *can,* but they prefer you to stop the immunosuppressive drugs *if at all possible* so the vaccine can work. When I asked my rheumatologist what to do, he said it was up to me. I decided that a risk of an autoimmune flare was smaller than the risk of dying from rabies if the vaccination didn't take, so I discontinued the use of CellCept for three weeks.

I made it through twenty-one days before I showed any signs of a flare, and the flare was only in my skin that time. I got back on the CellCept, and my skin responded quickly to going back on the medication. I looked at this whole episode as a blessing in disguise: my body held its own for three weeks without the main immunosuppressant, and upon re-starting the medicine, it worked immediately. Proof that my remission was holding strong. Better yet, the blood tests showed I had built up immunity to rabies, just as I should from the vaccine.

Unfortunately, the hits kept coming. I'm embarrassed each time I have to tell people I'm sick; it gets repetitive and just seems so unreal. When I cancel plans due to illness the person on the other end invariably asks incredulously, "Again?"

Yes, again.

Will Science Connect the Dots?

A week into Batageddon, I got walking pneumonia. It sounds ridiculous for someone to get pneumonia in May, but there it was: probably from a spring cold or allergies. The good news was I was off CellCept when I got pneumonia, so my antibiotics worked in record time for me. Round one of antibiotics cleared up an infection for the first time in years.

Hopefully science will catch up with reality soon and connect the dots between all of the ailments that seem like they should be related. Once they find the connections, it should be easier to manage them. Wouldn't twenty symptoms being part of one disease be a lot easier to understand than one person having twenty separate and distinct illnesses?

Creative Tips for Empowering Yourself

- Find humor in bad situations: draw a picture, write a poem, cry, scream out loud, punch a pillow—do something to express and release your feelings.

- Realize that we as patients can affect change in the medical world. Write letters to your congressperson requesting more research; join the Muscular Dystrophy Association, Myositis Association, and any other organization that represents your condition. Share your story. With more information, the medical community will have a greater chance of seeing the connections.

- Sharing my story, including the humorous points of views, has been cathartic and empowering. Share your story, too, so that others will know they are not alone; you will help yourself while helping them realize their own strengths. You can blog, join or create social media sites, journal, write letters, and speak up at your support groups.

- Repeat after me: "By focusing on being productive and helping other people, I step out of my own pain and end up helping myself."

Caregiver Tips

- When your loved one breaks down and "loses it," know you don't have to solve the problem. Your loved one wants to be heard, to be held, and to have a chance to let it out.

- Continute to love even when your loved one is weak.

Create Your Own Marvelous Transformation

It's time to grab your journal and spend a few minutes contemplating what you've read. Use the following prompts to guide you.

1. What situation or example resonated most with you in this chapter?

2. When faced with similar situations, how do you feel, act, or think?

3. What would you most like to remember from this chapter?

4. Going forward, how will you find humor in the least humorous of situations?

5. Review your three funniest and three most upsetting things that have happened due to your illness. Write down something you can learn from each of the humorous situations. Then, write something humorous for each of the most upsetting ones.

6. Think about how you can find gratitude for the little victories in life. Write down three things you are grateful for in this moment.

7. If you've never been to or considered counseling as a way to cope with your illness and its attendant stresses, write down your top three reasons why (as in, why you haven't done it or considered it). Now, write down three ways in which counseling could be helpful to you.

8. Finally, look back at the notes you made before you read the chapter. What changes do you notice in your thoughts since then?

Chapter Seven

Love Handles, Moon Face, and Body Image

Take Stock of Where You Are Now

Make some notes in your journal before reading the chapter.

1. List the three things you like most about your body. Now write down the three things you like least. Describe how your medication and the illness changed what your body looks like from the outside.

2. Now, on a new page in your journal, compose a love letter to your body. Express what you love and appreciate about it, and how grateful you are for the hard work it does to deal with your illness. This may seem a little strange and awkward at first, but trust me, addressing your body directly will make you realize the truth of these assertions and help you release any

negative feelings you may be subconsciously punishing your body for.

3. Have you ever been in a situation where you felt out of control of your body image and got angry or sad? If so, how did you handle it? Write down what you felt in the moment, what you said to yourself, and whether it restricted any of your activities out of shame.

The Wonderful Pieces of Divinity
I Have Found

Your loved ones love you, all of you, unconditionally.

.

You can love yourself unconditionally, too.

.

Forgive yourself for not having the perfect body.

.

Be thankful that you can exercise.

I have spent the better part of my adulthood feeling out of control of my body—not only the health of my body but also my skin and my weight. I know many people with autoimmunity share this feeling.

My skin is usually red and inflamed. I do all the right things to protect it—avoiding harsh chemicals, wearing sun protective clothing and sunscreen—but I still end up with cherry red blossoms of blotchiness. My fingers have Gottron's papules; my nail beds are often broken and red; my face looks very dry with the heliotrope rash over my eyes; and my chest has so many broken capillaries that I look like I have polka dots. I also have the "V-sign" and the "Shawl sign"—rashes that look exactly like they sound. The V-sign is a rash on the chest that imitates sunburn after wearing a V-neck T-shirt. The Shawl sign is a rash spanning the back, as if you placed a lace shawl around your shoulders.

I can't shave my legs because when I do my skin breaks out in an itching nerve-pain rash that feels like fire ants were running up and down both extremities. I have little sores in my ears that bleed; I shed skin; and I lose a third to a half of my hair every winter.

I can't wax or pluck my eyebrows because I get huge bumps and scabs that last longer than any smooth arches would have lasted. About once a year someone convinces me that *they* know how to wax eyebrows without causing a rash. So once a year I end up with a three-month scab where I used to have hair.

I look distracted sometimes, staring into space, because my body always has some vibration or pulsating going on somewhere. At times it is so prevalent that it gets painful, distracts me from what I am doing, and so I zone out.

Your Body Will Act Like a Yo-Yo

When you are on and off medications—IVIG, prednisone, Plaquenil, methotrexate, CellCept, Quinacrine, Elavil, Trazadone, Ambien, Valtrex, various pain medications, anti-inflammatories, and antibiotics, as well as a host of over-the-counter (OTC) meds—your body acts like a yo-yo. Regardless of your diet and exercise regimen, your body weight will change to its own tune.

If you personally have autoimmunity, I bet you can recite this part with me from your own experience: Have a flare? Gain fifteen pounds. Take prednisone and initially lose the fifteen, only to have it replaced by another twenty pounds brought on by a different form of the same meds. Then, there is the bloating and the water weight. Some days I felt so bloated I thought my skin would tear open from the internal pressure. At one point it didn't matter how little I ate or how much I exercised, I just watched the scale go up, up, and away as I gained and gained and gained.

I am mindful not to react to this in front of my daughter because I don't want her to internalize body image issues. But it hurts to look in the mirror and see someone you don't know and realize you have no control.

My heaviest non-pregnant weight was 178 pounds, which, at my five foot two and a half inches, was extremely uncomfortable. I carry it in my face and neck—let's call it my "fneck" since they cease to be separate entities—and in my abdomen, around and into my back. Most people call this "moon face," when the face gets so swollen from prednisone that it gets round and flat.

On countless nights I cried myself to sleep because the bigger clothes I went out and bought for my "puffier days" wouldn't button. Despite my physical limitations, I try to maintain a fairly physical life—biking, hiking, walking, and jogging—and eating carefully to combat the meds—all to no avail.

I used to wish I could wear a sign that said, "I don't overeat! It's my medications that make me fat!" That's how ashamed I felt. I was so self-conscious I was convinced people were staring at me as I ate, judging me for every bite I took.

The Reaction I Hope You'll Receive

One day, during a dark moment, I looked at my naked, lumpy, red and pale-white, splotchy body in the mirror. What I saw was Jabba the Hutt. Autoimmunity affects everything, including and especially your sense of sexuality. It was just about stolen from me in that moment.

I looked at my husband. I told him how ugly I felt and asked how he could stand to look at me, much less touch me. I saw nothing desirable and couldn't imagine what he could see either.

His answer was a simple one of perfect and unconditional love. He put his arms around me as he explained that he loved me, and therefore, he desired me. He lovingly assured me that my body wasn't ugly; it had just changed. I was alive and not dead; I was his wife. Now stop criticizing yourself and come to bed.

As a significant other of a person with a chronic condition, know that this is the reaction we need when we feel at our lowest about our appearance. We need to be accepted for who we are in that moment, not for who you wish we would be, for who we used to be, or for who you think we could become on the outside if we worked just a little harder. There is no "harder." We are already working enough just to survive. The gift of acceptance is more powerful to your loved one than any medicine, magic elixir, or miracle treatment. It is the gift of unconditional love.

Body image is about how we see ourselves, so while Scott's words comforted me, they didn't remove my inner pain and turmoil. I had to find a way to love my own body, just the way it was, in the moment, for itself.

What You Say to Yourself Is Important

I changed my self-talk. I thought of the days when I could barely walk and felt grateful I was now able to walk for miles a day. My body became less a matter of looks and more a matter of what it was able to accomplish. I appreciated how hard my body was working to be as healthy as it was, instead of resenting it for being sick and swollen.

Degrading oneself silently is no less detrimental than saying it aloud, and I realized I had still been judging myself for something I had no control over. Here I had been working to stop wallowing in the unfairness of the disease, yet I had heaped a dose of self-inflicted unfairness on top of it: unfair self-judgment that had no place in my life whether I was healthy or sick.

I attempted to love my body as unconditionally as my husband and told it daily that I accepted it as it was. I wondered if the negative self-talk was, in fact, part of my problem. In directing anger at my body for its inadequacies, was I harming myself?

In his book, *The Hidden Messages in Water*, Masaru Emoto describes that crystals form in water in accordance to the words spoken to it. Was I hurting my body, or at least my own experience of my body, through negative self-talk? In reflecting on this and over a period of time, I was able to change my approach from just faking to my daughter that I loved my body just the way it was to actually *loving* my body, love handles and all.

Recently, things have changed. I came to realize that the two vices I had continued to indulge in—a twenty-six-year diet cola habit and an occasional fast food burger—were probably the worst choices I could make, given my condition. I gave up both, with the help of an acupuncturist in Medford, Oregon, and the Chinese medicinal herbs she prescribed. Not only do I feel great but the weight has fallen off like never before: I now weigh 130 pounds. While I was exercising and eating healthy, *except for my diet soda and an occasional fast food burger,* I had no idea how bad they really were for autoimmunity.

Fifteen years ago, health experts announced that aspartame, the artificial sweetener in diet sodas, had been linked to autoimmune diseases. I dismissed it at the time and had never been able to break that addiction. More recently, Yale came out with a study linking the high content of sodium in fast food to autoimmunity. As it turns out, my two vices were a double whammy for my disease.

It is possible that I'll have a flare in a month or in a year or in five years, and then I might gain all of the weight back. There are no guarantees. Meanwhile, I will enjoy being thinner for however long it lasts and deal with the future when it comes. I am choosing not to live my life in shame or in fear of it any more.

Creative Tips for Empowering Yourself

· Commit right now that you will give yourself unconditional love and acceptance. No more self-judgment.

· Stand in front of the mirror and take a moment to look into your own eyes. Repeat after me.

I love myself.

I love and accept my body.

I love the healing work my body does every day.

I grant myself permission to be who I am,
how I am, where I am—today.

I choose peace.

· Do this daily and eventually you will feel a change take place within you. You'll notice you'll start to believe the words you're saying. There will be a new bounce in your step and a smile on your face. With this mantra you can initiate and manifest a new inner understanding of your outer reality. You can learn to love your body and the way it looks even if it is different from how you wish it to be.

Caregiver Tips

- Be aware of, and sensitive to, the fact that in autoimmunity, body image takes a beating.

- Your greatest gift to your loved one is unconditional acceptance.

- Partners do not have to be enraptured with each other to the point of wanting to rip each other's clothes off like teenagers; being able to express true, deep desire and love, in spite of unwanted physical changes, is a beautiful spiritual and emotional gift. You didn't marry (or commit to) your partner's body—you committed to his or her soul, mind, and being. Always keep this spiritual perspective alive and physical limitations will become truly irrelevant.

Create Your Own Marvelous Transformation

Now let's reflect on what you just read. Use the following prompts and questions to guide you in integrating your new insights and deeper self-understanding.

1. What situation or example resonated most with you in this chapter?

2. When faced with similar situations, how do you feel, act, or think?

3. What would you most like to remember from this chapter?

4. I shared my darkest, lowest self-esteem moment in this chapter—in fact, I cry every time I reread it. Your journal is private, only for

you to see. Write down your deepest darkest memory related to your body image.

5. Now, write a new love letter to your body, just another page in the journal, incorporating your new understanding.

6. Look back at what you wrote at the beginning of this chapter. How have your thoughts and feelings changed after reading the chapter?

Chapter Eight

Adults Say the Darndest Things

Take Stock of Where You Are Now

Consider the following questions and respond to them in your journal.

1. How have people treated you regarding your health? Has your illness affected the way you are treated at work? At school? Do you receive support, understanding, and kindness? Do you find yourself on the receiving end of doubt or unsolicited advice? Note a handful of the experiences that come to mind, and then write about how they make you feel.

2. If you've ever had strangers make comments about your condition, how do you respond? What do you say to them?

The Wonderful Pieces of Divinity
I Have Found

You can speak up for yourself.

·

You have nothing to prove to anyone.

·

There is no reason to feel guilt or shame.
You are not at fault. Your disease is happening
in your body, but it is not who you are.

·

Pay no mind to the opinions of others;
they haven't lived your life.

·

Being open and honest with a partner
is a gift in many ways.

·

Listening to and honoring your body
and its limitations is not lazy; it's smart.

·

Your suffering has made you more
compassionate and patient with others
than you might otherwise have been.

Everyone has an opinion. Many people don't have filters or boundaries to know when it is appropriate to share those opinions. Some of my autoimmunity is invisible, but there are parts of it I have to wear outwardly, like the rash. Other things aren't as obvious until I tell a story or open my big mouth.

Don't You Know?

I spend the majority of the summer covered up with sun-protective clothing, hats, and scarves, and carrying umbrellas like I were going on an African safari, even though we live smack in the middle of the United States.

A couple of years ago I showed up at our health club's pool for the first time. It imagines itself to be somewhat of a country club. Here were all of these hot-bodied young things, walking around in their barely-there bikinis, when I walked out of the locker room, unashamedly "fnecked," wearing a long-sleeved swim shirt and dress, a big bucket hat, and enough sunscreen to clog the filters for a year. Judging by the looks I got you'd have thought I rode out there on a unicycle wearing a wedding dress, backflipping right into the pool.

No matter how careful I am when in the sun, I can't prevent me from having red splotches on my face, most of which are a combination of an internal reaction and heat rash rather than sunburn. One summer it got really bad. I was afraid of leaving the house because on each trip out, some version of the following episodes would occur.

I walk through a store, minding my own business, three-year-old daughter in the cart.

Stranger approaches, "Excuse me, have you heard of sunscreen?"

I look around. Surely she isn't talking to me. "Hmm?"

Stranger, emboldened, "I said, why don't you wear sunscreen? You look really burned."

The first fifteen times this happens I reply, "Uh, yes, I use sunscreen," and I walk away.

Some strangers follow me. "Obviously not, or your face wouldn't be so red!"

I get mad, feel trapped, but don't want to cause a scene. "Okay, thank you for your concern." I am now *running away*.

After the *fifteenth time*, I got markedly less polite.

Stranger approaches. "Hey, heard of sunscreen?"

"Yes, thank you, I have but—as if it's any of your business—it doesn't help because I have a potentially fatal autoimmune disease that attacks my skin and muscles, and what you see is my body burning from the inside out, not a sunburn. Anything else you'd like to ask?"

Stranger gets a stricken look on his face, remains speechless as I walk away.

I didn't want to make anyone uncomfortable, but I was tired of people I didn't know coming up to me making *me* feel uncomfortable—and having the audacity to confront me in front of my daughter and scare her. Some people dared to ask what kind of example I was being to her. I should have replied, "What kind of example are you setting for your child by accosting a stranger in a store about something that is none of your business?"

Don't Claim Others' Truth as Your Own

There was no other way to make people shut up and leave me alone. All I wanted was to be left alone and shop in peace like everyone else. Being nice didn't work; ignoring them didn't work; so I was left with no recourse but to be extremely direct; that worked.

I realize at least some of those people were coming from a place of love and compassion, however inelegantly it was conveyed. They saw a person with painful, red, angry skin, and worked up the courage to share their knowledge about sunscreen they mistakenly thought I lacked. They didn't mean to attack me and simply approached me in the spirit of wanting to help. But I was not in a place to receive it in a positive way; being already so frustrated with it myself, self-conscious, in pain, and having heard it all before so many times.

Don't Claim It!

A few years out of college I worked at an outpatient correctional treatment center for female drug offenders. While they were building a program around a so-called twelve-step program, the place became extremely religious. People shared their religious beliefs and opinions, whether you asked for them or not.

I was largely undiagnosed at the time but going through a rough patch of fatigue, muscle weakness, and pain. I called in sick one day, and the next day my supervisor—a sweet woman whose intentions I *think* were based on love—called me into her office to check on me. She wasn't satisfied with my vague initial answer. She had noticed a pattern to my absences and wanted more in-depth information. I told her my history and that I was just having a bad week, with what they were currently calling fibromyalgia.

My supervisor closed her eyes, threw her hands in the air, and began yelling at the top of her lungs. I must "denounce Satan," she shouted, because surely my "illness is his handiwork." She said I must "stand up," then and there, and proclaim that, "By Jesus' stripes (his scourge marks as per the Bible) I am healed." Never again was I to utter the words "I am sick," because by proclaiming (saying) it, I was claiming it, and inviting it into my body.

I politely declined, explaining my beliefs differed from hers, but thanked her for her concern, excused myself, and returned to my office to do my work. She kept yelling she would pray for me—to my back—as I scurried away.

Be Wary of Belief Systems

Conversations like the above don't help an ill person. They create shame and guilt. I was raised Catholic and was still practicing at the time. Her words, while of a different Christian viewpoint, made me wonder if she was right, whether I was just not spiritual enough, faithful enough, or loving God enough. Or worse yet: perhaps God didn't love *me* enough.

During a time when I was already full of fear about what was going wrong in my body, I was now afraid that I had somehow invited Satan into my life. Today I no longer believe that an entity named Satan exists, but back then those words held real power and caused great fear for me. It set me on a course of shame and guilt, neither of which were helpful to either my spirituality or my healing process.

Threads of these kinds of stories and judgments exist in many belief systems. Think of the parents who were charged with involuntary manslaughter because they refused to take their children to the doctor due to religious beliefs. New Age spirituality's idea that we create our own reality by thought alone is another example of a beautiful concept that turns into a dangerous notion due to misinterpretation and misapplication.

What Neale Donald Walsch helped me understand through his mentoring was that my attitude and beliefs are not the cause of my disease. They can affect only how I feel about it and how I interpret it. God, my body, and life itself, have not forsaken me. I am not being punished for some unknown thing I did, and I wasn't maliciously singled out to be hurt.

Collectively, we as a society have created an environment full of toxins that are poisoning our bodies. Pollutants in our air and water are inescapable. Our foods have chemicals and additives in them that have been shown to cause immune system reactions, and, in more extreme cases, diseases. The lack of whole fruits and vegetables in our diets has caused us to be nutritionally deficient, and over-farming has made the fruits and vegetables we do eat inferior to those our grandparents consumed.

I am not at fault for getting my disease and cannot simply wish the physical symptoms away. Understanding this has cleared the way for me to stop being angry—at myself, at my God, and at the world.

How Can You Treat Your Spouse Like That?

Chronic diseases can tear families apart. Scott and I have an amazing relationship in which we laugh and cry together as we go through the daily journey of life. I spend every day in gratitude that we found each other and that I get to share my life with him. He is supportive in ways I couldn't have imagined, even if I'd been asked to design the perfect mate.

He bears more than his share of the heavy lifting in our marriage. Whenever I mention that to him, he responds by telling me of the things I do to make our life beautiful, of the emotional support I lend to our family, and of the wonderful wife and mom he sees in me in spite of my disease. We have managed to make our marriage an equal partnership of love and acceptance.

However, be careful who you confide in about the day-to-day details of how your disease affects you. Someone I used to think was a friend once criticized me for being a selfish wife because I allowed my husband to do household chores after the hours he works. This "friend" scolded me for not having a piping hot dinner on the table when Scott walks in the door, and for not always being sexually available despite how sick I am. How dare I not choose to be the perfect 1950s Stepford wife?

This person wanted to know how I could treat my husband like I do and warned me that Scott would eventually grow to resent, unless I grew up and stopped whining about not feeling well. I was cautioned that if I didn't buck up, I would end up alone.

How anyone who knew even the most basic facts about my disease could say such things was a mystery to me, and profoundly disturbing. I was stunned and initially tried to defend myself until it became clear that my words were falling on deaf ears.

So I gave up.

Do You Find Yourself Scrutinized?

I relayed the conversation to Scott, who found it laughable, and we moved on. But it made me think how many other people with autoimmunity find their marital behavior scrutinized by friends with implicit and veiled threats that, unless you shape up, your spouse might leave you.

My friend may have been genuinely worried about the status of my marriage. However, there are nicer, less judgmental, and more tactful approaches to the subject.

Again? Really? Tell the Truth!

Not everyone's ideas and opinion are as outlandish as those of the previous example. Sometimes people say or do things that are hurtful when they really don't mean to be. I try not to take things personally because I know these comments and actions are not meant the way they come across. Let's face it—I have been known to speak out of turn myself.

We all judge ourselves harshly and we all, sick or not, have insecurities that we sometimes project onto others through our words. Judgment is detrimental, whether directed at yourself or others. Even when things are not always presented in the most loving manner, the intent is probably not to demean or hurt us. People generally have good intentions, but their meaning can get lost in translation.

The problem is that words hurt more when they hit too close to what we already think and fear about ourselves. When I get the fifth infection in a month and I'm already feeling ridiculous and a friend says, "Again? How can you be sick again?" It's crushing. I don't want to be sick again! I would do *anything* not to be sick again! Asking that question makes me feel like you suspect I walk around licking floors at the shopping mall, when in fact it's quite the opposite. I fantasize about borrowing NASA's decontamination room and wearing it when I go out in public.

What You Eat Is More Important than You Think

Many studies point to a link between autoimmunity and diet, and I can attest that the chemical ingredients in processed foods tend to aggravate my system, causing flares of my disease, along with migraines. Due to throat muscle and swallowing issues, I also have a really sensitive gag reflex. Over the years I've found that when I minimize my exposure to certain foods, especially processed foods, I feel much better.

To optimize my health and that of our family, we opt to eliminate gluten and eat mostly organic foods. Still, if something is overcooked, too soft, mushy or stringy, there are times when I just can't eat it, no matter good how it tastes. Numerous people have accused me of being too picky, obsessive, or that I'm just making it up. But it doesn't matter what other people think about how we choose to feed our family. What matters is that we are comfortable with our decisions.

Sometimes people's reactions to our limitations can be hurtful. When I say I can't do something, lift something, or go somewhere, I am honoring my body and assessing the risk of injury because I know if I slip and fall, the recovery will be too much to handle. I have heard things like, "Oh come on, just try harder" or "Stop being a wimp."

In an effort not to allow my disease to control *every* day of my life, I've made adjustments that allow me to choose what the disease affects and what it does not. That means I have to be very in-tune with my abilities and limitations on a daily basis.

For example, I love to cook healthy organic meals for my family, but on a bad day it's not so enjoyable. The muscles of my hands, arms, and shoulders have been attacked for so long that they are weak and deconditioned to the point that cooking can be a major undertaking. It is extremely frustrating not to be able to reach into the lower cabinet to lift the pots and pans. Opening jars or packages can be a challenge I'm unable to do alone; nor can I stir anything thicker than pancake batter. Grasping a knife can be hard at times and when I do cut or chop, my fingers hurt both inside and out. The mere act of holding my arms above a stove takes so much effort that by the time the meal is ready, it is difficult to carry the dishes to the table.

After homeschooling our daughter all day, taking her to the zoo or other activities, helping my nephew study for a test, and maybe even doing a load of laundry, cooking a meal can be the final straw: I am just exhausted. To the average person this may be inconceivable, but engaging in two or three activities in one day can really wipe me out.

I have to pick and choose the tasks to prioritize. If I overdo it, I will likely pay for it by nightfall, or at the latest by the following morning when I'll have trouble getting out of bed. It may seem lazy or indulgent that we eat a lot of take-out or go out for many meals. It's hard when you want to eat healthy, but we find it is possible by making better choices. These are simply adjustments we've had to make in order to address my limitations.

You Have a Right to Your Fatigue

Many have tried to find ways to describe just how tiring everyday activities can be. People with autoimmune disease and fibromyalgia suffer from fatigue that can be utterly devastating. A small task can deplete my energy for the rest of the day and even into the next. Do you experience similar things with your own daily chores? Are you frustrated by it?

I like to think of my daily energy as money in a bank account. I have a limited amount of money to use each day and, as my day progresses, I have to ration how much money (energy) I use for each task. When I'm out of money, I'm out of luck. There is no more, and I don't have any credit cards to borrow against to make it through the rest of the day. The most I can hope for is a nap to save some money for later. But even that doesn't guarantee I'll be able to save enough to make it through the rest of the day.

On many days I end up in bed watching TV by 8:00 P.M. because my body is so exhausted I can't move. However, due to insomnia my mind doesn't stop, so I lie awake until the morning hours, like a prisoner in my own body. I can't get up and do anything and can't get the rest I desperately need. As a result I start the next day with my account already in the negative.

For an interesting take on how chronic and autoimmune diseases like dermatomyositis and lupus affect daily energy levels, check out the "spoon theory" at ButYouDontLookSick.com. I found it through my online support group, and it's very descriptive—a great tool to help you describe to the people in your life your daily struggles with energy and fatigue.

What's most hurtful are the people who dismiss, ignore, and act like my disease doesn't exist. It's not the worst thing in the world, until they express that they can't believe I can't do something, or, even worse, when they accuse me of faking it to get attention. Trust, if ignoring the disease and pretending it didn't exist would make it go away, I would ignore it away. (I tried it once. It didn't end well.)

There are countless things I'd love to get attention for: my personality, my wit, my generosity, my loving parenting, my poetry—you name it. Creating a disease and taking toxic medications with harmful, often extremely uncomfortable, side effects is not one of them.

You Have a Right to Receive Attention

It is true that people who suffer from a disease ask for, deserve, and need the attention of their loved ones. Moral and physical support plays a vital role in their quality of life. Asking for help or simply stating that they can't do something is not a cry for attention; it is just that: asking for help.

Those who interpret our asking for help as something more sinister, like undue attention-seeking, have their own insecurities and are likely not even thinking about me when they react this way. They are reacting to their own stuff.

It is understandable that people want to minimize what others are going through: pain and suffering are uncomfortable to witness, and verbally reducing them is often the only way someone feels they can help. As if by saying, "It's not that bad" or "It'll be okay," they can make it so. What people don't realize is that saying such things makes the person going through it feel undermined and unheard.

It is strange when all you want is to get better, but at the same time you have to prove how sick you are or defend yourself against accusations that it's "not that bad." It became an internal contradiction for me: While fighting to heal my body, I'm also trying to make people believe I'm sick! The latter can take on an undue importance because we get tired of having our every move questioned and our feelings invalidated.

These opposing ideas about who I was in relation to the disease—"I am getting better" and "I have to prove how sick I am so they accept it and stop minimizing my pain"—left me confused and unable to focus my energy on getting better. I was stuck between two different ways of defining and representing myself to others: Trying to heal and change my mind about being sick, and attempting to prove I *was* sick.

It's most disconcerting to have people throw my actions in my face from one day to the next or from one hour to the next. For example, some people have seen me on long bike rides with my family and afterward accuse me of being selectively lazy when I can't unload the dishwasher or clean without frequent breaks (if at all). It's hard to explain that the muscles, strength, and endurance used are different for each activity. Riding a bike takes large muscles with fluid movements while unloading the dishwasher, sweeping the floor, or folding laundry take smaller muscles with more fine-tuned, repetitive movements. Bending over and getting up and down while cleaning has me winded, in pain, and wiped out within a few minutes, while a five mile bike ride leaves me tired and sore but rejuvenated.

The point is that hidden diseases are hard to deal with because most of the time people look at you and think you seem normal. Therefore, they assume you can do everything they can do, and when you cannot, they assume you are faking, being lazy, or simply not trying.

Release Your Need to Self-Validate

Letting go of the need to validate my disease to others was a big step in healing me emotionally. Most of it came down to knowing that the people who mattered most in my life—my husband, my family, my closest friends—all knew what I was going through and all supported me. I didn't need to prove anything, didn't need the approval of others, and didn't need people to acknowledge or even accept my illness to make my symptoms real. I knew the truth. I knew I wasn't lazy or faking it. I also knew I was doing everything I could possibly do to get better.

Being on the receiving end of many such misguided comments, I've learned a lot about compassion. I am slower to jump to conclusions about why someone else might or might not do something a certain way. I make fewer assumptions about other people's health and abilities. Above all, I have more patience with others because I never know what the other person might be dealing with.

Creative Tips for Empowering Yourself

- Other people's opinions are just that, their opinions. Don't try to justify or prove yourself to others.

- You didn't do anything wrong and the disease is not a reflection on you, a punishment, or an indication of who you are. Sit with this and allow it to sink in. You are not responsible for being sick. You are only accountable going forward, for how you live your life in response to the illness.

- Repeat after me: "I lovingly dismiss the voices and opinions of others. I stand tall knowing I have done nothing wrong. I control my interpretation of the situation and thereby my reality, even when I cannot control my physical limitations."

Caregiver Tips

- Be supportive of your loved one in word and action, both in private and in public. Other people take cues from you about how to treat your loved one. If they see you doubting or ridiculing his or her weaknesses, they will think it's okay for them to do the same. If they see you supporting and caring for your loved one, they will understand that that is how your loved one deserves to be treated.

- Be aware of your expectations. People with autoimmunity have limited amounts of energy and their reserves often run out more quickly than they anticipate. Be cognizant that the end of energy can sneak up quickly, and without warning, and that it frustrates your loved one as much, if not more, as it does you. Have an escape plan ready.

Create Your Own Marvelous Transformation

It's time to grab your journal and spend a few minutes contemplating what you just read.

1. What situation or example resonated most with you in this chapter?

2. When faced with similar situations how do you feel, act, or think?

3. What would you most like to remember from this chapter?

4. If you've ever lost it with a stranger, think back to that experience and describe how you feel about it now.

5. What can you do, going forward, to stop yourself from internalizing other people's opinions of you and your situation? Come up with a few simple, straightforward strategies and word them in a declarative, memorable way for your own future reference. For example, "I will not . . . ," or "If this happens I will . . ."

6. List the tools you now have that help you stop needing to validate your disease to others.

7. Finally, take a look at the notes you made before you read the chapter. How have your thoughts changed?

Chapter Nine

Seeing the World in Technicolor

Take Stock of Where You Are Now

Think about the following questions and respond to each prompt in your journal.

1. What gifts has autoimmunity given you? What positive things have you seen, understood, and/or experienced that you might not have had you been completely well?

2. Either draw a picture, write a poem, or simply jot down some notes to describe what your disease looks like in your mind. Try to find a way to capture how you represent its essence to yourself.

3. Now that you're looking at a clear visual image or stark description of your illness, write down the greatest loss it has imposed on you.

What is the biggest or most important thing you have lost due to your disease?

The Wonderful Pieces of Divinity
I Have Found

Your disease helps you slow down and live life fully.

·

Learn to smile through the pain.

·

The world is a beautiful place
when you allow yourself the time to look around.

·

Art, music, and poetry
are wonderful avenues for healing.

·

Don't be afraid of death, but allow being faced with it
to help you appreciate life on a new level.

·

If you have children, chances are you are a better parent
because of your disease. It makes you more patient,
a better listener, and makes you mindful
to take the time to enjoy your children more.

·

Don't be afraid to say, "I love you" when you feel it.

Be grateful for every moment you have on this earth.

As an overachieving, formerly shy girl, I have laser-like focus on my objectives. I can submerge myself in the task before me and forget the rest of the world exists. While I'm a great multi-tasker, sometimes I'm so absent-minded that I don't know what day of the week, date, or even what month it is.

If the universe didn't have other plans and I had been physically healthy, I might have become a career thrill seeker: one of those trial lawyers on CNN, representing high profile criminal defendants everyone loves to hate, or an FBI forensic psychologist jetting from city to city, tracking and profiling serial murderers on television.

I couldn't imagine sitting still, so I sought challenges at every turn and craved the adrenaline rush working in a dangerous career would provide. I was driven, and those two were the actual career paths I was considering as I studied psychology in my second year of college—right before everything changed.

It's not that I never had any fun; my fun was just often overshadowed with thoughts of what I was going to do later: the homework I had to do, my plans for the future, my worries about how to get there, and an obsession with the rules so that I wouldn't screw it all up. Living in the moment was really hard for me.

I wasn't mentally unstable. I was just wound up *really* tight.

Take a Breath and Look Around

I *was* an overachiever in every aspect of my life: Read faster than anyone I knew—check; got the high school job as a bank teller—check; got good grades—mostly check; got into my college of choice—check; got good college grades—check; achieved a complete personality makeover upon arriving in college—check. Even when I partied, I had to do it right.

When the first signs of illness hit and I was forced to slow down, unable to function at the level at which I was accustomed, I had to take a deep breath and look around. What I saw was astonishing to me. There was a whole world outside my books and my carefully laid plans. Colors turned vibrant, water sparkled, and the leaves on the trees fluttered. Each moment took on deeper meaning, and connections with other people became especially important.

I have always been a happy person. Louis Armstrong's "What a Wonderful World" is a natural soundtrack to my life. My parents nicknamed me "Sunshine" because even when I got into trouble, they'd end up laughing because I would smile even as I got told off.

I thought it was silly to walk around being sad because life was so much fun. Even as I got older and became sick, I maintained that disposition most of the time. The nurses in emergency rooms often comment on my smile and good mood, even as I writhe in pain. My answer is always, "There isn't much else to do but smile. It wouldn't change anything for me to do any differently."

I love poetry and music, and I've always been drawn to art. As my world changed and I began to value every moment for itself, it seemed each word I heard meant more, every note was sweeter, and every picture evoked more emotion. I became more present as a result, determined to enjoy life and all it had to offer.

I picked up a paintbrush, bought myself a guitar, played the piano, and wrote more poetry than ever before. Seeing and appreciating beauty wasn't enough anymore—I wanted to merge with it. I wanted to experience beauty, to create and express it. In doing so, I found a kind of peace I'd never known before. I'm not a proficient guitar player or pianist by any means, but to create music, however elementary, with my own fingers was therapeutic. Watching my art transform, from private reflections on my pain and love to illustrations in my children's books, was an amazing process.

Seeing the world in vivid color became a literal metaphor, as I filled my space with paintings and colorful accents. I was no longer afraid of expressing myself, no longer afraid of what other people would think. I pierced my nose and got pink stripes in my hair. I surrounded myself with colors and materials that made me feel good and happy.

Can You Be Okay with Sharing Feelings?

Our society doesn't encourage uninhibited expression of feelings. When I understood I might not live as long as I'd wanted, I threw that repression off and decided to *feel* without hesitation. People I love would never doubt how I feel about them. I would give and not be afraid of rejection, expressing my love freely without expectation of having it returned.

I no longer hide behind stoicism. I now weep openly with happiness, having removed the walls around my heart. Some people comment they've never had anyone say "I love you" as openly as I do. That means I am accomplishing my goal of living and loving openly and without restraint.

Although I wasn't a mom before I had autoimmunity, I believe it has made me a better parent. Being present in the moment and cherishing the beauty of life unfolding allows me to experience my daughter in ways I wouldn't have otherwise. Since I've always been aware of the preciousness of the moments I have with her, I treasure them differently than I might have if I'd felt they were unlimited.

Her laughter permeates my soul; her smile lights my heart. I listen to her nonsensical jokes with an interest now that I may have lacked had I not slowed down. I make sure to smell her hair when I hug her and never miss a chance to kiss her nose. We go for walks and take our time as we stop to look at flowers, caterpillars, and the leaves on the trees. We allow life to move at a slower pace as we enjoy each other.

I held her as an infant and stared at her features, soaking her in and memorizing everything about her, trying to imprint her image on my soul. I thought, "If this is all I ever have with her, I will make it count."

That is how I have lived much of my life. Not in fear—that would have been giving in to defeat—but in gratitude for every moment. I chose to walk through life drinking in every detail, smiling even when I hurt, and saying "I love you" without hesitation.

Creative Tips for Empowering Yourself

- Find something you are passionate about—your family, art, music, or nature—and embrace it. Let your passion be a lens through which you can absorb the beauty and vibrancy around you.

- Love deeply and completely. Tell someone today that you love him or her—without reservation or expectation that the sentiment will be returned.

- Repeat after me: "I have something beautiful inside me to contribute to the world."

Caregiver Tips

- Prepare yourself for new emotions and vibrancy as your loved one sees the world in new ways.

- You, too, can learn to love more freely and see the world more vividly.

Create Your Own Marvelous Transformation

Take your journal and use the following questions and prompts to assimilate what you are learning.

1. What situation or example resonated most with you in this chapter?

2. When faced with similar situations, how do you feel, act, or think?

3. What would you most like to remember from this chapter?

4. Having absorbed the message in this chapter, draw a new picture, write a new poem, or make a new set of notes to capture what your disease looks like in your mind. What is different?

5. As if you'd never made one before, write a new list of the gifts autoimmunity has given you. When you're done, compare it to the list you made before. Do you notice anything interesting?

6. Revisit what you wrote about your greatest loss due to your health. Think about it for a while, then look for the positive effects of this loss. The absence of one thing allows the presence of another. Describe what you ultimately gained as a result of your loss.

7. Once again look back at everything you wrote before you read the chapter, and compare it to your thoughts now. What has changed?

Chapter Ten

Sage

Take Stock of Where You Are Now

Think about the following questions and respond to each in your journal. If you don't have children, you can think about any other person whom you feel responsible for and take on a nurturing role. Much of what we experience with children can also be applied to our beloved pets.

1. How have your parenting experiences been changed due to your illness?

2. Does your child know the extent of your struggles? Does your child show signs of worrying? Describe any such signs.

3. What do you do to reassure your child?

4. Do you worry about your child's health because of yours?

If so, what are you most worried about? Provide as much detail as you can, as it will help your mind to see it on paper.

The Wonderful Pieces of Divinity
I Have Found

Children are our link to the divine.
Be grateful for each moment with your children.

.

Be grateful your children can communicate their fears
and you can listen to their concerns
and be present to them.

.

Autoimmunity can help you be a more present parent—
one of the greatest gifts.

.

Your children may be more compassionate having a
parent with autoimmunity.

.

Patience, patience, patience.

.

The little things in life are the most precious.

Parenting has so far been the single most enjoyable experience of my life. Dermatomyositis has added some challenges but also many pleasures. As I mentioned, I would not have chosen to be a stay-at-home mom if I were not dealing with an illness that made working impossible. I am grateful every day that I had a little push toward making that choice.

It has been wonderful to be able to be there for all of Sage's firsts, being a part of all the important moments of her life, seeing all her dance classes, skating lessons, practices, and events. I am blessed to be her biggest fan and her loudest cheerleader. I've been able to be there when she needed me, to comfort her when she was scared, to catch her when she fell, and to be the first one to kiss her boo-boos. There is nothing more fulfilling I could have done—no case I could have solved, no court I could have argued in—that could have topped being Sage's mom.

Having an autoimmune disease taught me that I don't always have the solutions to my problems in hand *right that minute.* I've become a far more patient person in general, and in turn, a more present parent. I realize that the things we get upset about are temporary, and life is much bigger than the little bumps in the road.

Rule Number One: Throw Out the Rules

We practice attachment parenting mixed with our spirituality, so we have very few rules in our house. One of them is that we treat each other with love in all circumstances, even when we are upset or angry. Another is that, as long as we are together and (relatively) healthy, we can handle anything. We don't get angry when something breaks; we clean up the messes together. We work together to create a home of harmony. This wouldn't have been my focus had it not been for autoimmunity.

I do get frustrated. One time Sage threw the ball inside the house for the fourteenth time and broke the infinity statue my husband bought me for our anniversary. Instead of getting angry, however, I paused and asked myself if she broke it on purpose. Since the answer is never "Yes," there is never a reason to get angry. She is seven years old and things are just things; they can be replaced. Her trust in my unconditional acceptance and love, on the other hand, is not something I can easily get back.

Being a child of a parent with an autoimmune disease is difficult. Sage is an attentive and intuitive child, and no amount of subterfuge works. She has watched me go through twelve surgeries and two extended rounds of IVIG that, even as they were healing my body, made me very sick. She traipsed along to doctor appointments, physical therapy appointments, lab tests, and to have x-rays.

She has seen me unable to move for fear of setting off the fireworks inside my head and unable to climb the stairs without gripping the railing. She has also seen me run six-mile jaunts. She knows when I don't feel well. I can try to pretend to be okay, but it never works. All she has to do is look at me.

She hears me talk about what foods aggravate me and what foods help me. She knows what my strengths and weaknesses are. Even as Scott and I have tried to minimize the severity of the disease and the long-term meaning of it, she seems to know. She has indicated fear about my long-term prognosis and has even asked if I will die. Unfortunately, some of her fears about my health have become internalized into fears about her *own* health.

Step into Your Child's Experience

It must be scary to watch your mommy, whom you are very much alike, be sick and wonder if that means you will also become sick. Sage has become very health conscious, hoping to prevent herself from getting my disease. We work to help her understand that my genetics/biology and environment were specifically tailored to my getting this disease and that she is safe. We tell her about how she is made up of half of her daddy's strong genes that will keep her safe.

These are huge concepts for such a young mind to understand. It is heartbreaking for me, as a mother, to watch her struggle with all this. It's bad enough going through it yourself, but it's even harder to watch it affect your child's daily life. It's worse still to see how it affects her emotionally—the fear and trepidation that she might also become very sick.

Fortunately, Sage is articulate enough to be able to express her feelings and fears. As her parent it is my job to answer her questions as honestly as I can and supply her with the tools she needs to cope with her fears. The trick is not giving her so much information that it scares her, but by listening and comforting her about my health, assuring her that I will be okay, and that she will also be okay.

One of the gifts autoimmunity has given Sage, aside from having a more open, patient, and understanding parent, is that she, too, is more open and compassionate toward others. She came into the world with an open and loving heart—this is her innate personality. I watch how she looks at people who are hurting and notice how her ability to be empathic and care for others has been heightened—that she is expressing it well beyond her years. She wishes to give comfort, to support, and to just be there for people. She loves naturally and has a gift for bringing light and hope to any situation. I believe her gift is amplified by her experience as the daughter of a parent with autoimmunity.

Rickey, my nephew who lives with us, has had a similar experience. He worries about me, helps me when I'm weak, and has developed a compassion well beyond his years. He is starting his career as a Reiki practitioner and massage therapist, in part, because seeing my daily physical pain has solidified his desire to help and heal others.

If you have children in your life, you are likely to encounter similar experiences with them. What can you do to smooth out the rough times for your child and foster his or her loving qualities?

Creative Tips for Empowering Yourself

- Hug your children close.
- Realize you can't always protect your children from the truth of your disease, but you can reassure them that everything will be okay.

- Repeat after me: "While my health may affect my child's life, she has her own purpose in the world. I can support that purpose while at the same time giving her comfort."

Caregiver Tips

- Be aware of how your children are affected by your partner's autoimmunity. They may suffer pain, anguish, and emotional turmoil. Children can learn compassion and a deeper love if you allow them to express their fears without minimizing their negative feelings.

- Strive to create a childhood as normal as possible for your children. You, as the loved one, will have to pick up more than your fair share of rolling around on the floor and playing the rough and tumble games, especially when your partner is not feeling well.

- You cannot hide your partner's health problems from your children, but you *can* comfort them and tell them that this doesn't mean they'll have to face those same problems.

Create Your Own Marvelous Transformation

It's time to grab your journal and spend a few minutes contemplating what you just read.

1. What situation or example resonated most with you in this chapter?

2. When faced with similar situations, how do you feel, act, or think?

3. What would you most like to remember from this chapter?

4. Describe any positive outcomes in your child's behavior and capacities to empathize with others as a result of your disease.

5. Going forward, how will you protect your child from the negative feelings and fears of having an ill parent?

6. Look back at what you wrote at the start of the chapter. How are your thoughts different now?

Chapter Eleven

They've Always Got My Back

Take Stock of Where You Are Now

Consider the following questions and suggestions and respond to them in your journal.

1. What is it like for you to ask for help from others?

2. Describe any embarrassing situations you've experienced with others as a result of your disease. How did you feel at the time? How do you feel about those situations now?

3. In what ways do you feel supported? In what ways you feel alone?

4. Make a list of the core group of friends and family with whom you feel you can be completely honest. If you don't have anyone

who fits that description at this time, list the people with whom you wish you could develop such a relationship.

5. Describe something that has happened to you that was so mortifying you wouldn't tell your best friend or partner about it. Write it down in your journal.

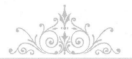

The Wonderful Pieces of Divinity I Have Found

Your family and friends will save you time and again.

·

Be grateful for the people in your life.

·

Showing love is a strength, not a weakness.

·

Autoimmunity can make you more passionate and sentimental.

·

Divinity is ever-present in your life through your family and friends.

When I love, I love wholeheartedly, and I have been lucky to find people who do the same. My triumphs over my disease are in many ways their triumphs because I would not be here today were it not for those people.

I want to share how these people support me, for two reasons:

1. To encourage you to find and appreciate these same wonderful support network in your own life.

2. To inspire you to allow people to support you if you aren't already doing so. Your family and friends most likely want to assist you; they may just not know how or they may be afraid to approach you for fear of violating your privacy or of making you feel inadequate.

Autoimmunity is isolating enough on the inside—it doesn't have to force you to walk through the world alone.

Use Your Most Valuable Resource

I recall hundreds of instances when our parents, family, and friends have come to our aid: The comforting calls when I am emotionally depleted, coming and taking care of Sage at all hours of the day or night, and helping us with household upkeep or warm meals. I've learned of new doctors, medical treatments, and alternative therapies because of their research. They keep me on my toes and don't allow me to give up, checking in on me and encouraging me to rededicate myself to self-care if I become lax. Their love, humor, and compassion bring a dimension of calm and levity to the most frightening moments.

Scott and I share our life, our hopes, our fears, and our good and bad days. Our experiences are so intertwined; he has not only supported me throughout but also suffered his own pain and stress as a result of my illness. He never accused me of hindering his career. Sometimes he doesn't make as many billable hours as he would like—I can tally up the number of hours he was at a hospital emergency room, doctor appointment, or at home tending to me when I am sick—and it's easy to see that. Whether he blames me or not, my health has put a considerable strain on his work.

Consider This About Your Spouse

There is another kind of emotional pain a spouse can experience, though it may be too taboo for them to talk about: the loss of a normal life. It would be really hard for Scott to admit this. Just as I have my breakdowns, my "it's not fair" days, he has to feel this way as well at times. He may be too selfless and concerned about me to voice it, or maybe even acknowledge it to himself.

It's not easy caring for me. Little things like unhooking my bra, fastening or unfastening buttons and snaps, putting on socks, washing or brushing my hair, or tying my shoes—all can become impossible for me, and he is there to assist. While he is doing them I wonder: did he really know he was choosing this life? At thirty-seven, did he envision himself having to dress his wife?

I imagine how hard it is to watch the person you love be in near-constant physical pain, get so sick from every germ, and fight so hard for a sense of normalcy—then to get well, only to be knocked back down unexpectedly. Every loving and protective instinct is activated, and yet there's nothing one can do except offer love and support.

Just as I shield our daughter from the realities of my condition, I do the same, although to a lesser extent, for Scott. This is due to my goal of enjoying life without reservation, to not live in fear, and to laugh through my pain, but also because I want to spare him. He bears so much for me, and I don't want him to carry more of the weight of my pain than he already does. If I can deal with it through meditating, smiling, joking, or bulldozing my way through my day, I will. There's no reason for us *both* to be miserable every time I am.

While writing this book, I asked Scott to tell me the truth about whether he has ever thought or felt the things I described. He hugged me and said, "Not really, because I don't know what any other life without you would be like." He has accepted our life without reservation on a level I cannot always achieve for myself.

You Gotta Be Okay with Embarrassment

The first time I developed shingles I was five months pregnant. I'd never had it before, and the doctors initially dismissed it as a rash that was part of my disease. I was on prednisone to prevent my body from rejecting the pregnancy, and it may have made the shingles worse or masked some of the symptoms.

The outbreak got really bad before it was finally diagnosed. One night I was at home with an oozing rash on my back when I awoke with nausea, severe stomach upset, and cramping. I ran to the bathroom yelling for Scott to come help me because I was in so much pain I was afraid pre-term labor had set in.

Scott walked in to witness projectile emissions from both ends. After it subsided *he* cleaned it all up and took me to the emergency room. Turns out the rash was shingles, and it was on a nerve pathway to the digestive system leading to the emissions along with dangerous dehydration. I spent the next few days in isolation in the hospital where they figured everything out and got me stabilized. Sage was born safely and healthy four months later.

Saturday Night Live used to have a skit called "Oops! I Crapped My Pants." That night in the ER, we calmed our fears that we were losing our baby by reciting lines from that skit. Humor got us through a dark, dark night. Seven years on and we still laugh about Scott having to clean up after my real-life, "Oops! I Crapped My Pants" episode.

In 2010, after a few months of IVIG, I was again having trouble with my digestion. The pre-meds I took to prevent the nausea and surges of motion sickness during infusions, along with my migraine medications, had led to three weeks of constipation. It snuck up on me. As my life began returning to normal thanks to the IVIG, I failed to notice I wasn't going to the bathroom.

After three weeks the constipation became an impaction with spasms. I tried all the home remedies, which only made it worse. At around 10:00 P.M., a dear friend offered to take me to the ER so that Scott could stay home with Sage. There I was, once again on my way to the hospital, with Mom on her way to meet us there.

The doctor determined that I did indeed have an impaction and gave me a cottonseed enema. I was in one of those ER rooms that have glass doors to separate you from the rest of the hallway. There was a curtain dividing the room, to give patients the illusion of privacy from their own visitors, if desired. There we were, Mom and my friend sitting next to me while I was lying down, waiting for the cottonseed to work. And then it did.

I was scared to be by myself because it hurt so badly. Being the great mom and friend that they are, they agreed to stay in the room, just on the other side of the curtain, as I used the portable commode and emptied myself into what looked like a popcorn bucket.

They had a wonderful time laughing, gagging, and threatening to post an audio recording of my moaning on social media. I was having less fun. When the doctor came to release me later he said it took a lot to impress ER nurses, but I had pulled it off by the sheer fact I had filled the popcorn bucket and then some. It was a proud moment right there.

We didn't eat out of popcorn buckets at movies for a long time after that.

I will quit while I am ahead; just know there are a lot more stories where those came from. I share them not for shock value, but to make two important points: One, when people are on your side, they will stick by you no matter what. This is unconditional love. Two, I want others with autoimmunity to know they are not alone in their embarrassing moments. They happen to all of us.

If you feel ashamed you're allowing the disease to control you, so don't. There's no need.

By letting you witness those two most uncivilized moments of my life, I hope you will feel that you, too, can live through having your loved ones experience them with you. You don't ever have to face scary or embarrassing experiences alone.

Your Opportunity: Choose Joy

It may be hard to believe after all I've shared, but my life and relationships aren't all about my disease. I am a nut and often make people laugh. I'm a klutz; I sing (a lot); I act like a child; I sometimes leave my common sense at home; and I have a big mouth. I think I am funny even when my friends, family, and others don't agree.

I choose joy and strive to make others feel cherished and to help them forget their own worries whenever I can. I love to live in the moment. Life is fun, and I intend to keep living it that way.

I have the privilege of calling a great number of people my friends. My life is rich with love, light, and laughter, due largely to the people who come in and out of it. Divinity abounds in my relationships, and I see oneness and connectedness in the way we can be apart and then pick up right where we left off.

You probably have relationships like these in your life. Pull those people close, cherish those relationships, and allow them to hold you up when you don't have the energy to do it for yourself. You'll be glad you did.

Creative Tips for Empowering Yourself

- Make a list of those you trust and can rely on for emotional support.

- Write a handwritten thank you note to each of those people—a heartfelt sentiment of appreciation letting them know what their help means to you. Send the letters in the mail. It feels wonderful to express your gratitude in this way to the people who have helped you the most. They, too, will feel good knowing what their actions mean to you on a deeper level than a verbal thank you could convey.

- If you currently don't have a strong support system, there is no time like the present: decide today to create one. Look around you and think about the people in your life on which you *could* rely. Choose one person from your family or friends and reach out to them. It could be as simple as calling that person and saying, "I am going through a rough health patch right now and could really use a confidante. This book I'm reading suggested I ask a friend (or family member) if they'd be willing to be my sounding board as I deal with my disease. Would you be that person for me?" Just having someone to talk to will be a big relief.

- Do the research and join a support group.

- Repeat after me: "Things aren't as scary when someone has my back. I can count on people in my support system to be there for me. I don't have to go through this alone."

Caregiver Tips

- Know you are your loved one's backbone. Going through this is bad enough; going through it alone is unimaginable.

- Autoimmunity can get messy. Accepting your loved one's embarrassing experiences with grace will help him or her feel safe. It is essential for your loved one to feel supported, especially in the most mortifying of situations.

- Be patient and understanding when your loved one can't do simple tasks. When he or she asks for help with something like getting dressed, it only takes a second for you to help, but it saves your loved one a lot of struggle and pain.

Create Your Own Marvelous Transformation

Time to grab your journal and spend a few minutes digesting what you just read. Let the following questions and prompts guide you.

1. What situation or example resonated most with you in this chapter?

2. When faced with similar situations, how do you feel, act, or think?

3. What would you most like to remember from this chapter?

4. Review your description of the most mortifying experience you can remember. Come up with three reasons why you don't

need to be embarrassed about it. Now consider the possibility of telling one person. It doesn't have to be today, but just the act of considering it will help to shine a new light on the situation, making you more able to laugh about it and to not feel so ashamed.

5. Finally, look back at your notes from the beginning of the chapter. How have your thoughts changed?

Chapter Twelve

Downward-Facing Dog

Take Stock of Where You Are Now

Consider and respond to the following questions.

1. What, for you, is the difference between *dealing* with illness, and *suffering from* it?

2. Take a look at your spiritual, religious, or faith-based beliefs. Consider what they mean to you, how you practice them, and what kind of comfort they provide for you. How, if at all, have they helped you deal with your illness in the past? If you've never applied them to your disease, why not? Or, if you have, in what ways can you expand on that application?

The Wonderful Pieces of Divinity
I Have Found

Autoimmunity can lead you to spirituality and yoga,
which lead to peace.

·

Yoga can help you be a better parent.

·

Suffering is a state of mind.

·

You can handle anything when you *just breathe*.
Spiritual fulfillment starts with passion and purpose.

·

Be more compassionate toward others.

·

Live a life of love.

My spiritual journey has been twofold: an intellectual unfolding through reading books, such as *Conversations with God*, *The Power of Now*, *The Four Agreements*, and *The Seven Spiritual Laws of Success*, and a physical-spiritual unfolding through yoga and meditation.

Through reading I found spiritual concepts that resonated with my core and helped me in understanding my disease. The notion that "you create your own reality" guided me to control my reactions to my disease even when I cannot control my body. Through my yoga practice I found peace and acceptance. Eventually, I wove the two together to create my yoga life.

I had been interested in yoga for a while but didn't take my first class until after I was diagnosed. In 2004 I received acupuncture treatments and practiced yoga at the same time. Through regular acupuncture visits, Chinese herbal medicine, and yoga, I was able to go off all immunosuppressant medications for a long time. They were also instrumental in my successful pregnancy.

As I became a mom the frequency of visits to my acupuncturist dwindled, and so did the status of my health. I had less time to spend having needles sticking out of me to balance my chi and less time to devote to yoga practice. I discovered, however, that the spiritual growth I'd gained through yoga had permeated my life, so that I was now *living* yoga mindfulness rather than just practicing it as an exercise.

According to Eknath Easwaran's translation of *The Bhagavad Gita*, the "higher mind—detached, unruffled, self-controlled"— is a state of "natural harmony that comes with unity of purpose, character, and desire. Negative states of mind do still come up . . . but there is no need to act on them."

I took this to mean that when I make a decision about who I am and how I exhibit that in the world, I cannot be affected by wandering thoughts or fears. I have the presence of mind and calmness to let such thoughts wash over and through me without penetrating or affecting my world. This is my yoga state of mind: mindfulness without pain, attention without judgment, presence without expectation, and no attachment to results.

A Beautiful Practice That Makes Your Struggles Disappear

Once I let go of the picture of what life should look like, and what I thought a *normal* life should be, I began to embrace life as it presented itself. It was a beautiful thing; my internal struggles disappeared—not my health issues, but the emotional struggles surrounding my health. My mantra is *just breathe*. It keeps me grounded and stops me from getting caught up in the drama of the moment.

It is a daily practice, much like yoga, and there are days when I, for some reason or another, choose not to practice it. Some days I'm depressed, angry, and filled with feelings about unfairness, judging myself for my limitations, and questioning if I've made it all up. I go through my catalog of scars and mentally pick at the scabs. Nevertheless, I've learned that even on those days, I can find moments in which I can choose to be happy, lighthearted, and grateful.

No matter what this day brings, tomorrow I can wake up fresh and ask myself newly who I want to be that day. I can choose to embrace life fully again, to inhabit my higher mind, and to eschew my emotional pain for the day.

Yoga mindfulness lets me enjoy my daughter more, appreciate my husband more, and better understand my parents. I can be kinder to others, embrace the silence, be more grateful, and have more patience. When I am off course on these things, I noticed I've usually stopped breathing—well of course I'm still breathing, but I mean I have stopped *breathing.*

Sage and I do this wonderful practice at night. In yoga, an instructor and his or her students will begin and end their sessions with a bow and an exchange of the word *namaste.* It means "the light or God that resides in me honors the light or God that resides in you." Sage and I started sharing *namaste* at bedtime to assuage her fears of being alone. Now she knows that even when she is in her bed, she is never really *alone* because we are connected through this light.

It was something she could grasp and hold onto at a very young age, and it was of great comfort to her. I shared this practice in my first children's book, *It's a Beautiful Day for Yoga*, in which a family experiences a day of yoga, opening and closing the day with a loving *namaste.*

How You Can Make Struggle and Suffering Disappear

Moments of reflection and observing life without judgment are yoga's gift. When my sweet daughter doesn't want to sleep in her bed, rather than become angry, I listen with love, and my yoga life gives me an answer.

Living a yoga life—a mindful, calm, centered existence— allows me to walk around in a state of love most of the time. In the past I would experience intense bouts of road rage: I would honk my horn, flip off, and curse at other drivers when they cut me off. Now I try to put myself in the other person's shoes. I ask, "What if his wife's in the hospital, and he's trying to get to her?" I assume the other person has a reason for being erratic. I take a deep breath and go on without honking or raising a middle finger. When at times I still say a choice word, my back seat parrot is sure to point out when I've stumbled, and I'm getting better at that part every day.

When I strive to have "unity of purpose, character, and desire," I am much happier. My physical symptoms don't go away, but they don't affect me as much. Suffering ceases, and instead I focus on how to best cope with the stresses that accompany my disease. The sense of struggle disappears as I realize I can and will handle whatever comes my way. I meet any obstacles with a positive attitude. That is the gift that yoga has brought into my life.

When I live life fully—my purpose—I keep my actions, ethics, and attitude in alignment with that goal, and by keeping my eye on the bigger picture—remembering my goal is to be happy—I can accomplish anything despite my disease. I just have to remember that for things to be beautiful, they don't have to turn out exactly like I planned them.

Yoga is the spiritual path that has worked for me, but it doesn't have to be the one for you. There are many paths to spiritual fulfillment. What's important in beating the mental aspect of autoimmunity is that you reach inside and find your center, your purpose, and your inner stillness. Also know that, sometimes, the most unexpected outcomes are the best.

Creative Tips for Empowering Yourself

- Practice some form of meditation or prayer to refresh your spirit, quiet your mind, and soothe your body. You can start right now. Sit comfortably, take a deep breath, close your eyes, and quiet your mind. Imagine a waterfall: see the flowing, foaming water, hear the crashing sounds, feel the cool mist, smell the earth, and allow your body to rock and sway with the waves. Match your breathing to the rhythm of the water. If your thoughts drift to other topics, say "Ohm," as you stay mindful of only the waterfall. Sit quietly for a few minutes, inviting peace and calmness to enter your mind and body through your breath. If you feel called to do so, you can repeat a mantra, such as "I am one with the earth; I am safe and happy." You can also stay silent or keep saying "Ohm."

- Consider trying yoga or another low impact stretching exercise like tai chi. While they are physical activities, they help center the mind, body, and spirit for overall wellness.

- Learn to live in the moment: let go of attachment to results by enjoying the process of your experiences without the need to control their outcome. Enjoy your experiences as they unfold, knowing they will turn out perfectly in the end.

- Find or define your "unity of purpose, character, and desire." Ask yourself, "Who do I wish to be?" Based on your answer, you can then align your actions, ethics, and attitude with your goals.

- Repeat after me: "I don't have to suffer. Suffering is a state of mind. I can choose happiness. I can accomplish anything when I put my mind to it."

Caregiver Tips

- Consider being involved in your loved one's exploration of his or her inner self. Being clear about, and connected to, this purpose helps your loved one stay focused on health instead of illness. You can be instrumental in that journey.

- Be open to joining your loved one for a yoga class or attending self-development classes or spirituality workshops with him or her.

Create Your Own Marvelous Transformation

Use the following questions and prompts to guide you in solidifying your insights and tracking your transformation.

1. What situation or example resonated most with you in this chapter?

2. When faced with similar situations how do you feel, act, or think?

3. What would you most like to remember from this chapter?

4. Where do you look for, and find, your own inner stillness? Describe what it looks like, sounds like, feels like, tastes like, and even smells like when you are calm and centered.

5. How do you quiet that voice inside when you want to be still? As you take a moment to go inward, and you notice that thoughts are flying through your head, how do you address them? Consider writing down any repetitive thoughts in your journal. Sometimes they just want to be heard and noticed, which you can do by writing them down. Don't get angry or frustrated. Acknowledge them, thank them for their presence and input, and then let them go.

6. Come up with a name for your inner calm, the space or place where your higher self resides. I call mine my "Yoga Life." Acknowledging it in such a profound way as naming it will help you stay true to who you wish to be. Keep in mind that your path (and the name of your inner calm) can change. Nothing has to be set in stone.

7. By identifying yourself by your inner calm and higher self, you quiet your internal skeptic (the voice that tells you what you can and cannot do) and transcend your physical circumstances. Write down in clear, simple language your response to the question, "Who do I wish to be today?"

8. Look back at what you wrote before you read this chapter. How have your thoughts changed?

Chapter Thirteen

I No Longer Fear Death, Nor Am I Inviting It In

Take Stock of Where You Are Now

Consider the following questions and respond to them in your journal.

1. Describe your thoughts and feelings about the things you've been told about the mortality rate and chances of recovery from your condition. Do the statistics scare you? What have you done to date to deal with these fears?

2. Do your doctors bring up concerns about malignancies, organ failure, and death? If so, how do you feel when they do?

The Wonderful Pieces of Divinity
I Have Found

Death need not scare you.

·

You are here to stay!

·

Awareness of mortality helps you live in the present
and appreciate life.

Have you experienced those feelings of impending doom, such
as wondering, *Will this be my last vacation? Will this be my last
birthday?* Or *What if I don't see my child's eighteenth birthday?*

We receive many mixed messages about whether our disease
is fatal. Prognosis numbers range from having five years to live to
the prospect of complete remission—there is just no way to know.
Everybody reacts differently to the disease, and it's impossible to
generalize.

I have the juvenile form of dermatomyositis, with a mortality rate
that is substantially lower than the adult-onset form. But truthfully,
they really *don't know.* The medical profession's understanding of this
disease is quite recent, and while advances have been made, there isn't
a lot of hard scientific information out there. That has not prevented

the discussion with nearly every specialist I've had from turning to the subject of death. It's usually innocent enough, and often implicit:

- Methotrexate (or CellCept) decreases mortality rates but carries its own risks of death.

- IVIG will lengthen your life span.

- You need to use sun protection every day if you want to see your daughter grow up.

- The incidence of cancer is XYZ. Have you had your cancer screening, colonoscopy, trans-vaginal ultrasound, and lung x-ray yet?

- Why have you never been tested for X (insert unpronounceable string of syllables)? It is very prevalent and very dangerous!

- You need to have this blood work done to check for cancer markers. It costs $750. It will tell us if you have cancer starting to form anywhere in your body. (Insurance declines to pay for the procedure, so I never had it done. Talk about anxiety.)

- You appear to have developed a rare and serious bacterial infection. Have you visited the tropics lately? Within the same hour, week, or a month later: "Oops, our mistake, you don't have it."

- It's up to you whether to continue taking the immunosuppressant medications while you get the rabies vaccine: it might lower the vaccine's effectiveness. Good luck!

Who wouldn't be scared? I've lived the past two decades with the specter of death hanging over me, whether the threats were real or not.

Trite? Perhaps, but True

Attitude has everything to do with how you feel. It's not how *sick* you are but how you *feel about it*. All the coping mechanisms I've discussed—humor, embracing one's family and friends, enjoying the little things in life, concentrating on one's children, taking up art— have kept me in such a positive attitude that I have not succumbed to the disease.

While attitude cannot change the physical realities of the disease, it did affect whether or not I was overcome by it. I constantly find new things to live for, which makes me fight and never give up. During the times when I retreated and said I've had enough, I got worse, my body stopped fighting, and things started to go downhill.

When I'm in a positive mood, smiling through my tears, and holding my husband, nephew, and daughter as tightly as I can, I take my meds more faithfully and seek out new treatments. I would go so far as to say that when I'm happy and emotionally open to life, my body seems to accept and utilize my treatments more effectively.

Am I afraid of death? No, from a spiritual perspective, I'm not. I think of death as a beautiful rebirth that is pure bliss. I feel that my soul will have a chance to be reenergized and released from the pain of this disease. Each instance of human existence is but a blip on the whole of eternity—I have no fear about the end of this life.

If I were to die tomorrow, I would have lived a happy, fulfilled life. I wouldn't have left anything unsaid or undone on the spiritual plane.

Having said that, I'm *not* ready to leave this earth. No matter how accepting and evolved I feel about death itself, I'm still a mother with a small child. The thought of how my death would affect her helps me know that death is not an option: giving up can't be a part of my vocabulary, and rest is a long way off.

The support system I have in place would take incredible care of Sage and make sure she was okay in the event of the unthinkable happening. Her life would go on, beautifully and perfectly.

However, I am not ready to leave Scott, Rickey, or my daughter. I have so much more to do here. I have so much more to share, more flowers to smell, hugs to give, and "I love you's" to say. Sage gives me strength, the drive to push on, encouragement to laugh through the pain and tears, and to fight harder than ever before. I plan on being here for a long time yet to watch my daughter grow up.

So, no, I'm not afraid of death. But I'm not inviting it either. I'm far from finished here.

Be Sure You Have a Plan

I now have a wonderful treatment plan that combines both Western and Eastern medicine, and I'm feeling better than I have in a long time. I'm stronger, eating healthier, and sleeping better. These are good indicators that I'll be around to embarrass and pester my family and friends for years to come.

Glimpses of mortality have made me appreciate life on a deeper level as I learn to live in the moment. Hugs touch my soul, flowers smell more fragrant, colors are more vibrant, and love-making feels more passionate. I haven't gone sky-diving or Rocky Mountain climbing like Tim McGraw's song suggests, but I do live like I'm dying—and it is magnificent!

Creative Tips for Empowering Yourself

- Smell a flower, watch a sunset, nuzzle your child's neck, and say "I love you." These things will fill you with joy and peace and will make today brighter.

- Don't dwell on what might be. Make a decision right now that you'll move forward enjoying all that life has to offer.

- Repeat after me: "Yesterday is over and tomorrow will take care of itself. This moment is all there is. I will make the best of it!"

Caregiver Tips

- When your loved one gets scared, just listen. Don't feed into it and don't let it affect your own peace of mind. When your loved one is afraid, he or she just wants to feel heard.

- Assure your loved one that, while you don't expect him or her to go anywhere, you will take care of the children and will handle all the other things he or she is concerned about if it were to happen.

Giving your loved one peace of mind does not encourage him or her to stop fighting but allows the worrying about death to stop and the business of living to continue.

Create Your Own Marvelous Transformation

Use the following questions and prompts to help you integrate any new information you've gleaned, and create a new sense of mastery over the issues touched on in this chapter.

1. What situation or example resonated most with you in this chapter?

2. When faced with similar situations, how do you feel, act, or think?

3. What would you most like to remember from this chapter?

4. What will you do to view death and, most importantly, your opportunity to live life fully, differently?

5. What will you do to maintain your hope and joy and not get caught up in fear of dying?

6. Look back at what you wrote about the things doctors talk about that scare you. Consider each example, and try to look at each dire warning as nothing but an invitation to take good care of yourself. Come up with three to four ways in which you can turn your fears into a positive action or a positive attitude today. For example, if you wrote, "my doctor keeps testing for cancer," you could write to replace that fear with: "my doctor is on top of the testing, and we will catch any changes early."

7. Draw a picture of your body in your journal. Then draw whatever symbolizes love, happiness, and health to you (a big heart, smiley face, flower, etc.) right on top of your body. The more elaborate, colorful, and happy the better. Now tear the page out of your journal, kiss it, fold it up nicely and put it in your purse or wallet. No matter where you are, any time you feel down, defeated, or scared about the future, pull out this page and see yourself safe, happy, and full of life.

8. Write your body a thank you note. For example, you could say, "Thank you for taking care of what we are dealing with right now. Thank you for how hard you work to keep us safe. Thank you for doing your job."

9. Look back at what you wrote before you read the chapter. How have your thoughts and feelings changed?

Chapter Fourteen

The Disease Does Not Define You

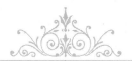

The Wonderful Pieces of Divinity
I Have Found

Autoimmunity is insidious and insistent. It infiltrates every
aspect of your life and inserts itself into every moment.
It's up to you to say, "No, you do *not* define me!"
By standing firm with the things that *do* define you
there's no room left for the other stuff. By looking for those
things that fill you with love and strength in your life,
you will harness your inner power to fight your disease.

Creative Tips for Empowering Yourself

The following is a list of activities and themes we've discussed so far that contribute to a spiritually balanced and happy life despite autoimmunity. I encourage you to take your notebook or journal and reflect on each one in turn, noting down what it means to you. Think about how you already have and/or how you can increase space and time for each of these pieces of divinity in your life. The goal is for you to articulate and thereby fully realize the power you have over your life and your state of mind. At the end of your reflections you'll be able to say: "Take *that*, autoimmunity! You may have control over my immune system, but you will never control my reality."

- Practicing gratitude and acceptance

- Enjoying life

- Trusting myself

- Trusting my support system

- Accepting unconditional love

- Finding strength

- Using humor

- Having patience

- Feeling compassion

- Seeking peace

- Giving love fearlessly

- Identifying purpose

- Releasing my fears about death so I can live for today

- Creating my own reality

One Final Task

Here's one final assignment for you. As we've discussed, your disease doesn't have to rob you of the good and the wonderful, the joyful, and the meaningful aspects of life. On the contrary, it can be the impetus that throws open the doors to more of those positive experiences. I invite you to take a moment and think about your new perspective. Can you now find instances of this positivity in your life? Have you perhaps learned a new way to interpret the events around you in a more positive light?

In your journal, create your own list of ways in which you can continue to reach for happiness. The first step is simple: just pick up your pen.

When you take control of your life by embracing these ideas, you will find the same peace and mental well-being I've found. You will know that you don't have to *suffer* because of your disease. When you align all parts of your self with the knowledge that, while you can't control the disease, you *can* choose happiness, all suffering and struggle dissolve.

No one *deserves* to be sick. Sickness is the result of what happens when your body reacts to toxins in the environment. Knowing this can release a lot of pain, guilt, and shame. You can stop feeling guilty about not being able to control your health. Dismiss any notion that your health is some kind of karmic punishment or lack of love from your god.

Creating my own reality means that even when I feel like a failure, I have in fact been controlling my interpretation of the disease and of the world all along. Through the wonderful pieces I have found, I've been expressing the highest form of myself, the part of me that at one with divinity. In that way, I have succeeded in beating my disease.

I will continue to fight, and I will continue to have bad days. Armed with my new knowledge, I know that no matter how bad it gets, I will have already won because I will have found the best part of my autoimmunity: I will have found myself.

Chapter Fifteen

Reality Check

I was able to come off of all medications in early 2014 and reached my lowest weight of 130 pounds. We had an active summer: a family vacation with a Disney cruise and trip to Walt Disney World, visitors from out of town, and plenty of other activities. I felt great. Most of the time I stayed healthy and strong, managing to avoid any sun exposure on our vacation and over the summer through the use of hats, sleeves, and scarves. I used natural herbs, vitamins, and oils for support and completed a month of paleo autoimmune protocol (AIP) to further cleanse my body.

All was well with my health and my world, and I believed it would stay that way. But things don't always turn out the way we hope. After everything I've shared about keeping a positive attitude, the following events plunged me into a bout of negative emotions—shame, anger, defeat, sadness, grief, and helplessness.

Wrap Me Up in Bubble Wrap

It was the middle of November when I decided to go skating with Scott, our daughter, and some friends. I took all of five forward strokes, stopped to talk for a moment, and then found myself inexplicably off my feet with my back on the ice. Our friend said my head hitting the ground sounded like a bowling ball falling on concrete. It felt that way, too. I had fallen so quickly that I'd made no effort to brace myself, flail my arms, or correct for the fall, and so my head hit with the force of my entire body.

When I woke up the next morning, I had all the classic signs of a concussion: nausea, dizziness, and disorientation. We went to Urgent Care, did a CT of my head, and found that all was well with the exception of a minor concussion and a strained neck.

The following February, I sprained my ankle while dancing at a charity event. I lost my balance and my ankle just gave out, my body crumpling around it. A trip to Urgent Care showed a sprain but no break. I went through weeks of unsteadiness and discomfort.

These are just a couple of my falls during the year, but I fall all the time. I fall down the steps; I trip over nothing in the yard; and I stumble if I am trying to carry anything over five pounds. I realized I needed to walk with more precision. I can't walk and chew gum at the same time: I need to concentrate and make sure every step is solidly executed. When I'm tired my falls are worse. One time after walking into a grocery store I was too exhausted to complete my shopping. I gave in and asked my doctor for a disabled placard for my car to conserve energy.

These injuries, and other minor ones, alarmed my family and friends. They noticed my lack of a startle reflex when falling and my inability to brace myself for impact. I was having increasing difficulty lifting anything heavier than a few pounds. I could barely open door knobs and jars. I couldn't go to the grocery store unless Scott or my nephew were home to bring the groceries into the house. Everyone hounded me to go to the doctor—they were afraid the next fall would be worse.

I asked my rheumatologist to see why I was falling (weakened muscles?), why I was losing mobility, and why I was unable to react (reflexes?). He recommended I get evaluated by a physiatrist (rehabilitation physician), who found severe weakness in my ankles and trunk muscles as well as deficiencies in my gait. He ordered gentle, isometric-focused aquatic therapy and had me fitted for a spring-loaded ankle brace. The brace didn't work, but the aquatic therapy helped. I didn't really see any increased strength, but my stamina was better, and we worked on correcting the problems with my gait. The latter turned out to be my coping mechanisms for weakness, which actually contributed to the worsening of my muscles. I have noticed more fluidity in my joints since I started therapy, which is increasing my stability and mobility.

Do My Eyes Deceive Me?

It was still in February when my rashes and shingles flared up. While treating them and looking to determine what was causing the outbreak, I noticed fogginess in my vision. One week I could see fine, the next I couldn't. I kept wiping my eyes, thinking they were overly watery; but nothing made my vision clear. The infectious disease doctor sent me back to my optometrist for a check-up: he was concerned the shingles had infiltrated my eyes.

It took the optometrist five seconds to find an opaque cataract in one eye and the beginning of one in the other; neither had been there at my last retina check-up a few weeks before. By the end of April, I'd had two cataract surgeries, an order processing for bifocals, and a huge headache. I couldn't accept that these eye problems were unrelated to dermatomyositis, and at last my doctor said there was probably a link. There was a chance they were a result of the repeated retina detachments, but more likely they were due to the long-term prednisone use or to a surge of my disease, as I had recently discontinued all immune system suppressants. Most likely of all, it was a combination of all of the above.

In between the staggered cataract implant surgeries, I walked and drove around with no depth perception. One day I rode up on the retaining wall in my driveway popping my tire. Another day, trying to get my car washed in one of those garage washes where you drive in and park between two rails, I couldn't point my car with enough precision to lace the rails. I got stuck, first with my tire on top of the rail and then, after spinning my tires on the wet pavement, I fishtailed my tiny hatchback and ended up at a sixty-degree angle from where I was supposed to be with the tire on the wrong side of the rail. My heart raced as I tried to remember the rules of being stuck. *Rock the tires* forward and backward. *Ease up* on the gas and then *punch it. Pray* with everything inside that I get out of there alive and without ramming my car into the sides. As my anxiety rose, so did my determination to get out. I gave it one last full throttle acceleration, turning the wheel the opposite direction from where my back end was going. When the car jumped back over the rail, I just kept going. I wanted to get away before they came to take me away. When I told Scott, and later that day my doctor, we decided I would not drive anymore until my eye treatment was completed, and I'd be able to get the correct glasses.

The summer continued in the same manner, and it was filled with tests: ultrasounds, pulmonary and cardiac function tests, more blood work, and multiple x-rays—all in the hope of ruling out the concurrent ailments and diseases that go with autoimmunity. Most of them were clear. My markers for active disease process were normal and continue to be so today. There were two exceptions: my white blood count (WBC) and a nodule on my thyroid.

The Words You Never Want to Hear

In July my rheumatologist was alarmed that my white blood count had not returned to normal even though I'd been off all suppressing medications since January. He homed in on a swollen, tender lymph node in my neck that had been there for ten years. He ordered an ultrasound and asked me to see the hematology oncologist, as a precaution, before I left Kansas City. It takes me four hours to drive from my home in St. Louis to Kansas City for my specialists, and I happened to be there alone, without my husband. Now I was faced with an oncologist appointment. I was scared.

Cancer was, for the first time in all my experiences with this disease, an actual possibility. When it was mentioned in the past, it was always a far-off concept, just checking to verify what we already knew, which was that it wasn't actually there. This was different. I was a wreck but kept telling everyone it was fine. Not once over the next three days, nor the following three weeks, while we waited for the results, did I utter the c-word, nor the l-word (leukemia).

A lady in scheduling—she was an angel, I'm sure—at Kansas University's Hematology-Oncology Center, took me under her wing and said to come to the clinic and sit there until she could convince someone to see me. She had one particular oncologist in mind. As I waited—keeping a cheery voice while telling Mom not to drive the one and a half hours from where she was for my *potential* appointment, and assuring Scott that I could handle it alone—what I really wanted to do was find a closet and curl up in a ball.

My scheduling angel did get me an appointment a few hours later. Sitting in the waiting area, surrounded by actual cancer patients, my resolve faltered. I became increasingly convinced that I had the c- or the l-word. I felt the fear and pain in the room, knowing that none of those people deserved it any more than I did. I decided it was inevitable: I would find out that I, too, had cancer.

Finally I met Dr. Yacoub, the hematology-oncologist. He was kind and thoughtful—willing to see me on his lunch break—

and surprisingly knowledgeable about autoimmunity, specifically dermatomyositis. He explained the blood work that had brought me to him (not too bad in his opinion); he explained the statistics of underlying malignancy being the cause of my disease (not high since I'd had dermatomyositis for so long). He also explained that dermatomyositis could have caused new malignancies to form, and while he was only marginally concerned (1 percent chance in his mind), it was enough to warrant sending me down the hall for a battery of blood work and then downstairs for an urgent CT of my entire torso. The urgency worried me. I came up with a new mantra and visualization: for the next couple of hours I repeated over and over, "My blood is clean and clear, it flows easily," while picturing little vacuum cleaners in my body cleaning up any errant cells.

Three days later, the first round of tests came back and the doctor called me personally to tell me that it was clear. He then went on to explain that we'd have to wait *three more weeks* for the final test, the one he was most interested in seeing—the one that, according to my mind, *would be positive*. He said "I believe there's only a 0.01 percent chance of it being positive. I'm being overly cautious by doing this test—most likely it will be negative—but with that result I'll be able to give you full assurance that you are cancer-free." This didn't reassure me. Scott and Mom, on the other hand, whooped with joy about this news.

Three weeks later Scott and I made the trip to Kansas City to receive the final results. In the waiting area I was on the verge of tears. Again I felt the pain, sadness, and fear of the people around me and became convinced it would be bad news. We held our breath as we walked into the room and listened to the doctor review the results. It took him thirty seconds to say that there were no bad results, that everything was clear, and that he was releasing me from his care indefinitely because there wasn't even one worrisome marker in all of the results. We didn't smile. Words were useless. We said thank you and left, unable to show emotion because we'd reached that level of depletion, mixed with relief.

When we got to the car, the dam finally broke. I cried and sobbed uncontrollably for several minutes, realizing how tightly I'd been bracing myself for those four weeks of waiting. At long last I could let it all go. I could return to a life without fear.

Stress Can Pull You Down, If You Let It

The stress of waiting for a cancer diagnosis (which thankfully never came) put my body on high alert and reduced energy. By the fall I was noticing a decrease in my strength and stamina and I got worried. Then one morning I couldn't lift my arms or bend my legs enough to put on my own socks. Despite my known adverse reactions to prednisone, I agreed to a rapidly declining dose, hoping it would reverse the weakening quickly.

It didn't. I felt even worse. Two weeks later we discontinued prednisone and restarted CellCept since I had done so well on it before. Within two months I gained twelve pounds, lost 20 percent of my hair, and found out my white blood cell count was again dangerously low—lower than before. Through conference among three of my specialists, it was agreed that IVIG was, again, my best option.

I was also told to see an endocrinologist as soon as I could for the small nodule on my thyroid. *Really?* I'd barely recovered from the last scare, decided to put that on the back burner for now, and pretend it wasn't happening. Denial was my friend in that moment because I needed to get my IVIG arranged.

Liquid Gold Runs Through My Veins Again

My infusions started out beautifully. I had no headache for the first three days, and I felt stronger by the minute. I received a healing touch treatment from a wonderful nun whom I'd known from previous visits. I took my pre-meds and didn't seem to need to take anything the rest of the day. I told my family this was the easiest IVIG experience yet. Then came the morning of day four.

I awoke at 4:00 A.M. with excruciating pounding, rushing sounds in my head, and a metallic taste in my mouth: I was having aseptic meningitis (AM) again, the IVIG allergic reaction. The slightest movement, sound, or deep breath sent me over the edge. Delirious, I thought, *My head is going to explode all over the wall. I hope Scott can get it clean.* I took pain and nausea meds and prayed for sleep.

Four hours later I woke up with the same symptoms, vomiting and dry-heaving for thirty minutes with a pounding headache. Scott was at work, so Rickey took over the reins. He called the doctor to see if I should still go to my infusion, all the while applying cold packs to my neck, giving me medicine, and massaging my head and shoulders. He also took care of Sage until her grandpa arrived. He handled the doctor's calls, kept Scott informed, and got me ready to leave when we got the news they'd set up an immediate hospital admission.

I was hospitalized for thirty hours, during which they pumped me full of antihistamines, pain and anti-nausea medicines, and a whole bunch of fluids. I was barely conscious enough to tell Sage good night on the phone. I was desperate for sleep but couldn't get comfortable in the hospital bed. Somehow I managed to drift off, and I woke up the next afternoon feeling lighter and free of the headache.

They released me with instructions to rest over the weekend and return to the infusion center on Monday to continue the infusions. We wanted to be better prepared this time and took our chances with an antihistamine, Periactin, that has been shown to help with reactions to blood products. It worked great! I had no headache for the final two days of infusions, and I continued to take it over the next few days for prevention. It was an exhausting few days, but I made it without any recurrence.

I'd Like to Teach the World to Sing

I used to have a natural singing voice. When I auditioned for a play in college, the voice teacher asked me to take lessons from him—I was surprised. I'd had no idea and no training. He said he could see I had talent but didn't know how to use it.

I took lessons for a few weeks but eventually got bored with it. I wanted to sleep and party instead. Then dermatomyositis stole my voice: made it ragged as it damaged my throat and vocal cords.

After my IVIG treatments were complete, Sage asked me what a certain song sounded like. Without thinking, I started singing it. My voice was so smooth and clear I hardly recognized it. There was no raggedness, no scratching, and it was coming out easily.

It was a reminder of how much this disease has changed my life and how many things I have lost because of it. I chose to be grateful for my treatment, grateful for my health insurance, grateful that I had a daughter to sing to, and grateful for the chance to have my singing voice back, even if only for a brief time.

From Here on Out

As I write this I'm waiting for an endocrinology appointment later this week, but I've decided to take back control of my reality and stop worrying about results. I have rediscovered my inner strength. I feel more like me again. It doesn't matter what the endocrinologist will say; like everything else, it will be okay, and even if it isn't okay I can make it mean whatever I desire. I was temporarily knocked off my balance by a succession of negative events, but I am back to myself again and will not let anything derail me, for right now.

My health, the health of anyone with a chronic condition, is a never-ending story of ups and downs. I was humbled to have many of my friends and family members comment on my strength and courage over this latest round of struggles, even when I didn't feel very strong or courageous at all.

That was the point of this final chapter: to share that even if we falter in our beliefs about ourselves and our health, even if we decide to give in, we can always change our minds again and return to our centered place—*in an instant*. That is what *The Marvelous Transformation* is all about. It is about being willing to be open and honest with yourself when you fall into old patterns and repeatedly inviting yourself to emerge stronger, without fear, and without hesitation. It is about forgiving yourself for being ill and forgiving yourself for having negative thoughts. It is about making a conscious choice to *live every day* that you are alive and not let the disease control you. As my experience has shown, we can traverse this whole process again and again and be continuously transformed.

Are you ready for your own marvelous transformation?

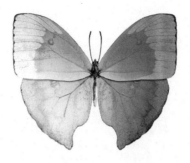

APPENDIX

Wonderful Products and Services I Have Found

In the nearly two decades that I have wrestled with this disease, I have tried many products and services to address my needs, both physical and emotional. It has taken a lot of trial and error to find things that work for me, and I want to share some of the best I found. If you are newly diagnosed, or just having trouble finding products that work for you, this section is for you.

Keep in mind that not all of these will work for everyone because we are all different and have various stages of a disease; but it is a starting point. I hope these will at least help you look in the right direction. Experiment to find out what works best for you. Even if none of these products and services work for you, I hope they will plant the seeds of ideas that will point you in the right direction.

Health and Beauty

LUSH Fresh Handmade Cosmetics

www.lush.com

LUSH promotes handmade cosmetics that utilize natural and organic ingredients. There are real fruits and vegetables in their products, and many of them are vegan. They minimize packaging (shampoo bars instead of bottles, for instance) and maintain a policy against animal cruelty. I have had so much trouble through the years with skin products causing skin reactions that I became very skittish about trying anything new even if it was labeled "natural" or "organic." When I lost half of my hair and had open bleeding sores, I walked into a LUSH store and begged for help.

They suggested I try their shampoo bar called *Soak and Float*, which is formulated for dry, itchy scalps and contains cade oil and lavender. They warned me that it would smell like a campfire, but I didn't care! I tried it, and my angry scalp calmed down within a week. I get four to five months of use from one shampoo bar because it only takes a quick swipe of the bar to make a whole lot of suds. I've also used their Veganese and American Cream conditioners, as well as their Sea Spray hair mist.

We use the bar soaps they offer for everyday hand washing—*Rock Star* is our favorite. I also routinely use *Dream Cream* for my face and body. When my facial rash is inflamed and painful, I can put *Dream Cream* on and within seconds the heat and pain subside. The lavender and chamomile have a real calming effect.

I have changed nearly all of my skin products over to LUSH with very few exceptions.

Some other LUSH items I love are: Dreamwash, Twilight Body Wash (only available during the holidays), Karma Kreme, their massage bars (solid lotion to carry with you for painful skin), bath bombs, and bubble bars. My husband and my daughter also use LUSH products, and we have turned many friends and family members into LUSHIES as well. It has definitely made a difference in the look and feel of my skin.

First Aid Beauty Skin Care Products

www.firstaidbeauty.com

A more recent find, First Aid Beauty skin care products has a line of redness-reducing creams and serums. I mix the Ultra Repair Cream and the Anti-Redness Serum and apply them together twice a day. They feel soft and smooth going on, and the effects, which are almost immediate, are amazing as the mixture calms my skin right before my eyes. They are allergen- and fragrance-free and are the first "cosmetic" facial lotions I've used without having a negative reaction.

Burt's Bees

www.burtsbees.com

I've had great success with Burt's Bees products. I use their spray deodorant, facial cleansing wipes, and lip balm. I've used their lotions as well.

Tom's Natural Toothpaste

www.tomsofmaine.com

Since I was cleaning up everything else I put on and in my body, I thought I'd try natural toothpaste as well. While I was afraid it wouldn't clean as well, my gums are actually much less sensitive since switching over, my teeth are just as clean, and my breath seems to stay fresher.

Sheer Cover Makeup

www.sheercover.com

I don't wear much makeup because it irritates my skin. However, when it was at its reddest, I felt I needed something to cover it. I used a mineral powder called Sheer Cover. At a time when my self-esteem was at its lowest, it helped restore my ability to feel pretty when I chose to dress up. It completely covered the redness and gave me the look of smooth skin. I didn't have any negative reaction.

Sun Protection

Being on immunosuppressant drugs, I'm supposed to wear sun protection every day of the year, rain or shine. I've tried every sunscreen, well, under the sun! The following are the sun protection products that have worked best for me.

EltaMD

www.eltamd.com

This is my favorite sunscreen. It goes on easily, doesn't clog my pores, doesn't make me itch or burn, and actually protects my sun-sensitive skin. It can only be purchased through a doctor, but the website has a physician finder. Ask your dermatologist if they carry EltaMD.

Vanicream

www.psico.com/products/sunscreens

I learned of this one from the Mayo Clinic and took that as a good recommendation. It works well, too, although I have had a bit more of a reaction with it than Elta, if not nearly as much as with department store brands.

Coolibar

www.coolibar.com

Sun protective clothing is a terrific way to decrease the amount of chemical sunscreens you use on your skin. I love Coolibar's products because they are soft and comfortable and don't make me hot, even in the hottest weather. In fact, I feel cooler in them than without them because they keep the sun's rays off of my skin. I've purchased jackets, swim shirts and skirts, scarves, neck gaiters, hats, T-shirts, and a sun umbrella. I have also outfitted my family with their products. My daughter even chose to have full-length swim pants because they were "so cute!" We've been happy with everything we purchased.

Headache, Pain, and Sinus Relief

Peppermint Headache Stick

www.epiphanyperfumeco.com

It looks like lip balm but goes on your forehead and temples. It's a natural aid in headache relief and while it doesn't conquer severe migraine pain, it does help with minor headaches.

Head Scratcher *(looks a little like a whisk with an open end)*

They are helpful in gently massaging the scalp and work best when someone else uses it on you.

Ice Packs and Microwaveable Heating Pads

These are some of my best friends. I alternate ice packs and heating pads on various parts of my body for many kinds of pain. Ice packs also help with migraines.

Essential Oils

We have been using organic lavender oil for years for relaxation and for support with mild discomfort. Young Living Essential Oils (100 percent pure organic essential oils) have changed my life. I use them to protect my body, calm myself in times of emotional distress, promote restful sleep, support proper joint and muscle function, alleviate minor pain and discomfort from headaches, support proper digestion, and maintain healthier skin.

I am so happy I found them and that my family has found benefit in them as well. While I hope to share my successes with you, please remember these results may not be typical. Check with your doctor for uses and drug interactions before trying any natural remedies.

Neti Pot for Nasal Irrigation

This is good for clearing sinuses, especially when used with sea salt and organic eucalyptus oil. I try to use this prior to OTC meds to work on sinus problems.

Food

We try to use all organic foods in order to maximize the nutrients we are giving our bodies. In our quest to eat clean foods, we have eliminated high fructose corn syrup and hydrogenated oils, as well as most other chemicals, preservatives, and additives from our home. Further, going gluten-free has produced good results. It can makes grocery shopping challenging at times, but the long-term effects on our health are worth it.

Eat Right for Your Blood Type
Book and website by Dr. Peter D'Adamo
www.dadamo.com

Food should nourish, support, and heal your body. Dr. D'Adamo's theory is that eating the proper food for your blood type helps your body take care of itself. I always crave red meat while my husband craves salads. When we were first dating, servers in restaurants would try to put my big fat juicy steak down in front of him and the dainty salad in front of me. I'd always feel slightly ashamed when I had to correct them until I found out that I have an O blood type (characteristic of meat eaters), and he has an A blood type (characteristic of veggie eaters). Seeing results from adopting a diet based on my blood type also confirmed that my body has been telling me what it needed all along—another reason to trust myself. The website above has information about the book as well as the various blood types and their recommended dietary requirements.

Grocery Delivery Services

Grocery shopping can present a challenge to people with autoimmunity for many reasons, such as pain, lack of energy, and the strength it takes to carry bags into the house. We recently started having fresh, organic produce and groceries delivered directly to our house via a company called *Green Bean Delivery*. This has minimized the amount of time and energy I have to expend on shopping trips, freeing me up to do and enjoy other things. The prices are comparable to our grocery store's local organic food section. There are many such services, and more popping up all the time. Check your local listings—you'll be glad you did!

Sleep and Music

White Noise Smartphone App

www.tmsoft.com/white-noise

I've been plagued by insomnia my whole life. A friend suggested I try this free app, and it really helped. I am able to fall asleep with more ease and sleep better throughout the night. It lets you to listen to nature noises, campfires, hairdryers, and a host of other soothing "white noise."

Music

Music relaxes, heals, and calms. Classical music is always a great choice, as are yoga and meditation soundtracks. One composer I want to recommend in particular is Elio. His music is designed to evoke specific emotions and healing frequencies, resulting in beautiful, rejuvenating, and relaxing pieces. I love his music so much that I partnered with him to compose music for the children's books I write. You can find out more about Elio's healing music at www.eliomusic.com.

Cleaning Products

With sensitive skin and any form of autoimmunity comes sensitivity to harmful chemicals and substances. Any harsh chemicals cause a problem for my skin, so we've sought and found natural alternatives.

I feel good about using these products because they are natural, non-toxic, and good for my health.

White Vinegar

I use white vinegar mixed with water in a spray bottle to clean and disinfect everything. It cuts through stains and mildew. It easily breaks up gummy, stuck-on stuff and works for everything. It is also cheap and safe for my skin.

Natural Detergents from Your Health Food Store

I have switched to natural laundry and dish detergent from our local health food store. I used to buy baby detergent but never thought about dish soap. The baby detergent was usually fine, but I did notice that my clothes would sometimes be irritating to me. Since switching to the natural detergents, I've had no more irritations from my clothing.

Second Medical Opinions

It's often advisable and necessary to seek further medical advice when your own medical doctors aren't getting anywhere. It's not unusual for patients with autoimmunity to travel for medical care. I certainly have in the past and am doing so now. In addition to the clinic and doctor recommended below, I've also heard good things about Johns Hopkins, but I haven't yet been there myself.

Mayo Clinic

www.mayoclinic.com

I turned to the Mayo Clinic at a time when I was getting nowhere with my local doctors. It was an expensive trip but crucial for me in getting on the road to better health. The Mayo Clinic is what got me started on IVIG treatments (my liquid gold).

If you're in a position where your medical care is not making you better, and if traveling is an option for you, the Mayo Clinic Department of Rheumatology is a choice I'd highly recommend. Keep in mind that there can be a long waiting list for Mayo's Rochester Clinic, so you might look at the Scottsdale (where I went) and Florida Clinics as other options.

Dr. Merhdad Maz, The University of Kansas Hospital

www.kumed.com/find-doctor/maz-mehrdad

Dr. Maz is my former Mayo Clinic doctor who is now in Kansas. If you live in or near Kansas City and are looking for a good rheumatologist, I highly recommend him. He is the doctor who prescribed the IVIG and got me on the successful path I'm on today. I was thrilled to find out he had moved within four hours of us, and he has once again taken over my care. I gladly travel the four hours to see him every couple of months—he's that good.

Alternative Services and Practitioners

Acupuncture

As I mentioned, for a long time I managed my disease with acupuncture and Chinese herbs. It is a viable option to consider if you find a good practitioner with experience and compassion. Acupuncture has helped me both emotionally and physically throughout the years. It has addressed my pain, my migraines, and even helped me have a successful pregnancy.

Some people worry that acupuncture is too expensive, and there is a movement called Community Acupuncture that endeavors to make the healing modality available to all people at a much lower rate by administering the treatments in a communal room. The People's Organization of Community Acupuncture has a list of participating clinics that can be found at www.pocacoop.com/clinics. To be listed, clinics must adhere to a voluntary sliding scale between $15 and $50, with $20 being the maximum for the low end of the scale.

Darby Valley, DAOM, LAC (Oregon)

Cottage Grove Community Acupuncture

www.cgca.us · Darby@valley.us

I was fortunate to have had Darby Valley, DAOM (Doctorate in Acupuncture and Oriental Medicine), LAC (Licensed Acupuncturist) for acupuncture and oriental medicine when he was in St. Louis. I credit his care for keeping my body happy and healthy and without medications for well over three years. He is one of the reasons I was able to carry my beautiful Sage to term. Here is a little note from Darby:

"For the last fifteen years I have used my training in Traditional Chinese Medicine (TCM) to help people maximize their quality of life. The combination of diet, exercise, meditation, acupuncture, and herbology is a wonderful way to make a difference. The nature of the practice of TCM on this continent is to be a 'jack of all trades.' I have worked as a family practitioner, with patients with autoimmune disorders, gynecology, geriatrics, infertility, and plain old everyday pain. I hope one day to open a traditional medicine inpatient facility to explore the full impact of traditional modalities in helping people heal."

Darby is currently practicing in Cottage Grove, Oregon. If you are lucky enough to find yourself near him consider paying him a visit.

Disclaimer: The process of getting off of my medications was carefully orchestrated and lengthy—not something to be taken lightly. Please consult with your acupuncturist and physician before changing any medications.

Nancy Burton, LAC (Oregon)

nancyburtonlac.blogspot.com · *(541) 646-0134*

Nancy treated me with acupuncture to comfort and give me hope. She also prescribed the Chinese medicinal herbs that assisted me in breaking my addiction to diet cola, as well as some herbs to aid in digestion. I credit her with starting the improvement in my health status. I've built upon her invaluable advice at home, and she continues to be a wonderful support system. If you find yourself near her, she is an amazing practitioner to check out.

Cori Scheitlin, Holistic Nutrition Consultant

www.good4thesol.com · *cori.scheitlin@yahoo.com*

Cori is my current nutritional partner in building my health plan. She is wonderfully supportive and insightful. She blends her knowledge of food, herbal supplements, vitamins and minerals to support the body's natural ability to heal its self. We work together to blend the nutrition and supplements with my Western medications to make an overall plan that ensures my ongoing health. Here are some thoughts she recently shared with me:

"Inflammation, such as a rash or pain, is not your body rebelling against you. It's actually working really hard for you. The body's ultimate goal is to heal and help you become aware of what is going on inside. We have been trained to think that physical ailments, especially pain, are bad because symptoms do not feel good. That makes us believe that our body is not working correctly, when actually, pain and ailments are a sign that the body is doing its job perfectly. It's releasing toxins, negative thought patterns that no longer serve us, and healing itself from the inside out. The body is alive and working hard to get back to homeostasis. Proper nutritional balance, supplementation with vitamins, minerals and medicinal herbs, can help support the body and encourage all body systems to work efficiently. There is a time and place for medications, and those shouldn't be ignored; with supplementation we can allow our bodies to work for us in conjunction with Western medications for optimal health."

Cori has helped me make a huge difference in my health, as well as my husband's. She offers a number of services, including online consultation for nutrition.

Massage Therapy

Massage therapy is another of my best resources. It makes a huge difference in my daily life. It not only relaxes and soothes the muscles that cause me so much pain, but it also assists in relaxing and uplifting my mind and spirit.

Support

A little research reveals a host of support groups and foundations for autoimmunity. I belong to a few Facebook support groups that have been very helpful: search for "Myositis Support and Understanding" on Facebook if you have myositis like me. I am a member of its board of directors.

Following is a list of resources—organizations, foundations, and associations—for people with autoimmune diseases and related disorders. Many of them are focused on specific diagnoses, but some are more general. They each have their own lists of resources that are worth exploring as well.

Autoimmune Disorders (General)

The American Autoimmune Related Diseases Association

Aarda.org

Johns Hopkins Autoimmune Disease Research Center

Autoimmune.pathology.jhmi.edu

The National Organization for Rare Disorders (NORD)

RareDiseases.org

National Institute of Arthritis and Musculoskeletal and Skin Diseases

Niams.nih.gov

PANDAS—Pediatric Autoimmune Neuropsychiatric
Disorders Associated with Streptococcus

PandasNetwork.org

Alopecia Areata

National Alopecia Areata Foundation

NAAF.org

ALS (Amyotrophic Lateral Sclerosis)

The ALS Association

ALS.org

Arthritis

Arthritis Foundation

Arthritis.org

National Institute of Arthritis and Musculoskeletal and Skin Diseases

Niams.nih.gov

Behcet's Disease

American Behcet's Disease Association

Behcets.com

Celiac Sprue Disease

Celiac.org

CeliacCentral.org

Crohn's and Colitis

Crohn's and Colitis Foundation

CCFA.org

Diabetes

DiabetesResearch.com

Diabetes.org

Fibromyalgia

National Fibromyalgia Association

Fmaware.org

Idiopathic Thrombocytopenic Purpura (ITP)

Platelet Disorder Support Association

PDSA.org

Lung Disease

American Lung Association

Lung.org

Lupus

Lupus Foundation of America

Lupus.org

Multiple Sclerosis

National Multiple Sclerosis Society

NationalMSSociety.org

Muscular Dystrophy

The Muscular Dystrophy Association

Mda.org

Myasthenia Gravis

Myasthenia Gravis Foundation of America

Myasthenia.org

Myositis

Cure JM (Juvenile Myositis)

CureJM.org

Johns Hopkins Myositis Center

HopkinsMyositis.org

The Myositis Association

Myositis.org

The Myositis Support and Understanding Association

Understandingmyositis.org

Psoriasis

National Psoriasis Foundation

Psoriasis.org

Sarcoidosis

Foundation for Sarcoidosis Research

StopSarcoidosis.org

Scleroderma

Scleroderma Foundation

Scleroderma.org

Sjögren's Syndrome

Sjögren's Syndrome Foundation

Sjogrens.org

Vasculitis

Vasculitis Foundation

VasculitisFoundation.org

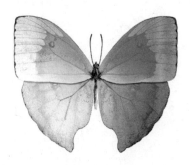

BIBLIOGRAPHY AND
SUGGESTED READING

*F*ollowing is a list of the books I mentioned, as well as additional books and other media I recommend for bringing about your own marvelous transformation. Some of them are inspirational and will make you think outside of your comfort zone; others will entertain you, make you laugh or cry, teach you about the world, and help you explore your inner landscape; many of them share stories about the triumph of the human spirit. Each of these books (and others by the same authors) has impacted who I am, how I view the world, how I relate to others, and, most importantly, how I manage my disease. I hope you will find your own joy, peace, and transformative wisdom within them.

On Inner Peace, Personal Growth, Spiritual Understanding, and the Resilience of the Human Spirit

Chopra, Deepak. *The Seven Spiritual Laws of Success: A Practical Guide to the Fulfillment of Your Dreams*. Novato: New World Library, 1994.

Claire, Em. *Silent, Sacred, Holy, Deepening Heart*. Ashland, OR: Emnin Books, 2009.

Coelho, Paulo. *The Alchemist*. New York: HarperOne, 1993.

Covey, Stephen R. *The 7 Habits of Highly Effective People: Powerful Lessons in Personal Change*. New York: Simon & Schuster, 1989.

De Becker, Gavin. *The Gift of Fear and Other Survival Signals that Protect Us From Violence*. New York: Random House, 1999.

Easwaran, Eknath, trans. *The Bhagavad Gita*. Tomales, CA: The Blue Mountain Center of Meditation, 2007.

Emoto, Masaru. *The Hidden Messages of Water*. Hillsboro, OR: Beyond Words Publishing, Inc., 2004.

Foundation for Inner Peace. *A Course In Miracles*. Mill Valley, CA: The Foundation for Inner Peace, 2007.

Hendricks, Gay. *Conscious Living: Finding Joy in the Real World*. New York: HarperCollins, 2000.

Hicks, Esther, and Jerry Hicks. *Ask and It Is Given: Learning to Manifest Your Desires*. Carlsbad, CA: Hay House, 2004.

Huber, Cheri. *Suffering Is Optional: Three Keys to Freedom and Joy*. Murphys, CA: Keep it Simple Books, 2000.

Johnson, Spencer. *Who Moved My Cheese?: An Amazing Way to Deal with Change in Your Work and in Your Life*. New York: G. P. Putnam's Sons, 1998.

Lipton, Bruce H. *The Biology of Belief: Unleashing the Power of Consciousness, Matter & Miracles*. Carlsbad, CA: Hay House, 2008.

Millman, Dan. *Way of the Peaceful Warrior: A Book That Changes Lives*. Tiburon, CA: H. J. Kramer, Inc., 1980.

Nhat Hanh, Thich. *Being Peace*. Berkeley: Parallax Press, 1987.

Redfield, James. *The Celestine Prophecy: An Adventure*. New York: Grand Central Publishing, 1997.

Riso, Don Richard, and Russ Hudson. *Personality Types: Using the Enneagram for Self-Discovery*. New York: Houghton Mifflin Company, 1996.

Ruiz, Don Miguel. *The Four Agreements: A Practical Guide to Personal Freedom*. San Rafael, CA: Amber-Allen Publishing, 1997.

Ruiz, Don Miguel, and Janet Mills. *The Mastery of Love: A Practical Guide to the Art of Relationship: A Toltec Wisdom*. San Rafael, CA: Amber-Allen Publishing Company, 1999.

Stein, Diane. *Essential Reiki: A Complete Guide to an Ancient Healing Art*. New York: Crossing Press, 1995.

Sui, Master Choa Kok. *Meditation on Twin Hearts with Self Pranic Healing*. Aquarian Visions, 2000. CD.

Tolle, Eckhart. *The Power of Now: A Guide to Spiritual Enlightenment*. Novato: New World Library, 1999.

————. *A New Earth: Awakening to Your Life's Purpose*. New York: Dutton, a member of Penguin Group, 2005.

Volo, Karin. *1,352 Days: An Inspirational Journey from Jail to Joy*. San Diego: Life With a Fabulous View, Inc., 2015.

Walsch, Neale Donald. *Conversations with God: An Uncommon Dialogue (Books 1–3)*. Charlottesville, VA: Hampton Roads Publishing, 1996–1998.

————. *Home with God: In a Life That Never Ends*. New York: Atria, a trademark of Simon & Schuster, 2006.

What the Bleep Do We Know? DVD. Directed by Betsy Chasse, Mark Vincente, and William Arntz. Starring Marlee Matlin and Elaine Hendrix. Goldwin Films, 2004.

On Relationships

Beattie, Melody. *Codependent No More: How to Stop Controlling Others and Start Caring for Yourself.* Center City, MN: Hazelden, 1986.

Bernstein, Albert. *Emotional Vampires: Dealing with People Who Drain You Dry.* 2nd ed. New York: McGraw-Hill, 2012.

Huang, Chungliang A. *Mentoring: The Tao of Giving and Receiving Wisdom.* New York: HarperCollins, 1995.

Keel, Philipp. *All About Us.* New York: Broadway Books, 2000.

Zukav, Gary. *The Seat of the Soul.* New York: Fireside, 1990.

———. *Spiritual Partnership: The Journey to Authentic Power.* New York: HarperOne, 2010.

For Parents, Children, and the Young at Heart

Dyer, Dr. Wayne W., and Kristina Tracy. *Incredible You! 10 Ways to Let Your Greatness Shine Through.* Carlsbad, CA: Hay House, 2005.

Filmore, Emily A. *It's a Beautiful Day for Yoga (With My Child Series).* Eureka, MO: Beautiful Day Publishing, 2009.

———. *It's a Beautiful Day for a Walk (With My Child Series).* Eureka, MO: Beautiful Day Publishing, 2009.

Howson, Susan. *Manifest Your Magnificence, Affirmation Cards.* Toronto: Magnificent Creations, 2002.

Munsch, Robert. *Love You Forever.* Willowdale, Ontario: Firefly Books, Ltd., 1986.

Sears, William, and Martha Sears. *The Attachment Parenting Book: A Commonsense Guide to Understanding and Nurturing Your Baby. New York:* Little, Brown and Company, 2001.

Thomas, Marlo. *Free to Be . . . You and Me.* Philadelphia: Running Press Kids, 2008.

Walsch, Neale Donald, Laurie Lankins Farley, and Emily A. Filmore. *Conversations with God for Parents.* Faber, VA: Rainbow Ridge Books, 2015.

Williams, Margery. *The Velveteen Rabbit.* New York: Doubleday, 1958.

For Cultural Understanding and/or Pure Enjoyment

Angelou, Maya. *I Know Why the Caged Bird Sings.* New York: Bantam Books, 1983.

Anthony, Piers. *On a Pale Horse (Incarnations of Immortality, Book 1).* New York: A Del Ray Book, Random House Publishing, 1983. (And the rest of the series)

Fey, Tina. *Bossypants*. New York: Little, Brown and Company, 2011.

Hurston, Zora Neale. *Their Eyes Were Watching God*. New York: HarperCollins, 2000.

Kingsolver, Barbara. *The Bean Trees*. New York: Harper and Row, 1988.

Lee, Harper. *To Kill a Mockingbird*. New York: Grand Central Publishing, 1960.

Neihardt, John G. *Black Elk Speaks: Being the Life Story of a Holy Man of the Oglala Sioux, The Premier Division*. Albany, Excelsior Press, an Imprint of SUNY Press, 2008.

Quinn, Daniel. *Ishmael: An Adventure of the Mind and Spirit*. New York: Bantam Books, 1993. (And the rest of the series)

Welty, Eudora. *Eudora Welty: Photographs*. Jackson, MS: University Press of Mississippi, 1993.

United Nations. *Universal Declaration of Human Rights*. Geneva: 1948. Available at: http://www.un.org/en/documents/udhr/.

Various Perspectives on Food and Health

D'Adamo, Peter J. *Eat Right 4 Your Type: The Individualized Diet Solution to Staying Healthy, Living Longer & Achieving Your Ideal Weight*. New York: G. P. Putnam's Sons, 1996.

Fuhrman, Joel. *Eat to Live: The Amazing Nutrient-Rich Program for Fast and Sustained Weight Loss.* New York: Little, Brown and Company, 2003.

Hay, Louise. *Heal Your Body: The Mental Causes for Physical Illness and the Metaphysical Way to Overcome Them.* Rev. ed. Carlsbad, CA: Hay House, 1988.

Hunt, Tate. *The Gluten-Free Bible,* Tate Hunt, Lincolnwood, IL: Publications International, 2010.

Life Science Publishers. *The Essential Oils Desk Reference.* 6th ed. Orem, UT: Life Science Publishers, 2014.

Trescott, Mickey. *The Autoimmune Paleo Cookbook: An Allergen-Free Approach to Managing Chronic Illness.* Seattle, WA: Trescott LLC, 2014.

Wahls, Terry. *The Wahls Protocol: A Radical New Way to Treat All Chronic Autoimmune Conditions Using Paleo Principles.* New York: Penguin, 2014.